An A-Z Guide to Food Additives

Never Eat What You Can't Pronounce

Deanna M. Minich, Ph.D., C.N.

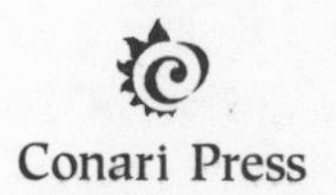

Conari Press

First published in 2009 by Conari Press,
an imprint of Red Wheel/Weiser, LLC
With offices at:
500 Third Street, Suite 230
San Francisco, CA 94107
www.redwheelweiser.com

ISBN: 978-1-57324-403-9
Library of Congress Cataloging-in-Publication Data available upon request.

Cover and interior design by Maija Tollefson
Typeset in Scala and Officina

Printed in Canada
TCP
10 9 8 7 6 5 4 3 2 1

The paper used in this publication meets the minimum requirements of the American National Standard for Information Sciences—Permanence of Paper for Printed Library Materials Z39.48-1992 (R1997).

To my sister, Brenda, and to all those who need assistance in finding their way among the massive explosion of processed foods in this age of fast living

Contents

Acknowledgments

Thanks to my mother, I was probably one of the few nine-year-olds in the 1970s who could read nutrition labels. After all, it isn't often that children are taught to understand words like "mono- and di-glycerides" and "BHT." Her brilliant insight and earnest quest for knowledge about the food supply started me down the path I walk today—sharing nutritional information with others is now my life's mission. My passion has been funneled into ensuring that people have the knowledge they need about foods to become and keep healthy. As I was writing this book and telling others about it, I was met with an overwhelming response to the idea of having this resource available. People are hungry for guidance on understanding the complicated food supply–I thank all of you for being the truth-seekers and continually questioning the quality of the foods you eat!

In my life, there have also been a number of other teachers and mentors who have passed on their nutritional pearls to whom I express heartfelt gratitude:

Phyllis Bowen, Maria Sapuntzakis, Henkjan Verkade, Roel Vonk, Barb Schiltz, and Jeffrey Bland.

My sincere thanks go to my amazing agent, Krista Goering, whose heart is embedded in the work of bringing health information to others. I couldn't ask for a more skilled, compassionate editor than Caroline Pincus, who has been an absolute delight to work with on this and other book projects. And, finally, I thank Mark and my three furry friends for their patience and support in the creation of this book.

Disclaimer

This book contains, to the best of the author's ability, accurate and current information, but it is not a comprehensive guide to all chemicals that exist in the food supply. The author and the publisher do not assume any liability for ways in which the information presented in the text is applied or interpreted, or for any loss, damage, or injury incurred by relying on information contained herein. This book is not intended to be a substitute for medical counseling and supervision, and is not for the purpose of diagnosing, treating, curing or preventing any disease. Please see a qualified health-care professional if you need medical advice.

Introduction

"If you can't pronounce it, don't buy it."
—**Elson M. Haas, MD,** author of *Staying Healthy with Nutrition*

"Don't eat anything your great grandmother wouldn't recognize as food."
—**Michael Pollan,** author of *In Defense of Food*

Our modern society has birthed a new language: Food Additive-ese. Unless you're a nutritionist, food technologist, or chemist, chances are you don't understand much of the new jargon, but you're immersed in it every time you go to a grocery store. Store shelves are laden with thousands of words waiting to be deciphered, and hundreds of new ones are piled on every year. This language, spoken on volumes of food labels, is speckled with infamous "unpronounceables"—long, polysyllabic, knotty, chemical-ized names of additives that have made their way into our everyday eating. Trying to speak this language is like talking with a mouthful of marbles—your speech becomes garbled and you end up spitting the word out with a winced face, accompanied by a shot of embarrassment and slight giggle.

To make life easier, food additives are now disguised with "code" names. Instead of tongue-tripping over their chemical names, you can now spout out their perky, friendly acronyms or brand names—BHA rather than "butylated hydroxyanisole" and aspartame in place of "aspartyl-phenylalanine-1-methyl ester." The complexity of the language and the hoops you need to jump through to translate its vocabulary make knowing what you are *truly* eating a tenuous venture.

Although food additives are often used in small amounts, these minute amounts add up. The average American consumes about 150 pounds of food additives a year, the bulk of it sugar and sweeteners, followed by salt, vitamins, flavors, colorings, and preservatives, representing almost 10 percent of the food we eat each year. To make choices you feel good about, you need an "additive translator" to help make sense of it all. With this book as a personal guide, you will be able to tiptoe through the field of additive landmines and ingredients that may cause allergic reactions like headaches, fatigue, and breathing difficulties, or those that cause you to get bloated or feel hyperactive.

> The average American consumes about 150 pounds of food additives a year, the bulk of it sugar and sweeteners, followed by salt, vitamins, flavors, colorings, and preservatives, representing almost 10 percent of the food we eat each year.

But let's back up a moment. While in the trenches at the supermarket, have you ever stopped mid-aisle to question how the food supply came to be complicated and convoluted to the point that you need an expert to tell you what to eat? Why should you need a book like this just to understand your every bite?

If we observe from a distance, we uncover a possible answer in our everyday frenzy. Day-to-day routines have become just a bit crazier, packed with extended working hours and overflowing with responsibilities. Our eyes and ears are bombarded with continuous, mind-numbing sound-bytes delivered by e-mail, radio, and TV. Technological advances are multiplying, renewing the flow of information every couple of hours. The only way to survive and succeed is to simplify. Nowadays, if we can't say something in six words or eat something in six bites, we may not be able to give it our undivided attention. One of the ways we have achieved our quest for convenience is at the expense of our nourishment. Packaged, ready-to-eat foods allow us to squeeze it all in—to be nothing less than "superhuman." In return for handy prepackaged edibles, we now need to learn "labelese" to make sense of it all. Ironic isn't it? We try our best to save time with convenient foods, but then spend extra time just learning what we are eating.

Thanks to food additives, packaged items can now sit on the shelves for years and be ready to eat whenever you are, if you have the patience to break through the casings of cardboard, Styrofoam, metal, and plastic. Additives give foods an internal "makeover" by improving their flavor and appearance and replacing nutrients lost in processing. Technically, they are defined by the Federal

Food, Drug, and Cosmetic Act set forth by the U.S. Food and Drug Administration (FDA) as any substance which becomes a part of the food matrix as a result of "producing, manufacturing, packing, processing, preparing, treating, packaging, transporting, or holding food; and including any source of radiation intended for any such use." With the average food traveling 1500 miles or more to your dinner table, you can only imagine the mosaic of food additives that have become a part of what you are eating.

> The FDA defines an additive as any substance which becomes a part of the food matrix as a result of "producing, manufacturing, packing, processing, preparing, treating, packaging, transporting, or holding food; and including any source of radiation intended for any such use."

Unless you grow your own foods, what you eat is beyond your immediate control. Consumers are at the whim of farmers, food industries, ingredient manufacturers, and supermarket buyers. Is there anyone looking out for you? The FDA has the job of overseeing food safety. Fortunately, with the advent of the Internet and accessible information, we are becoming more knowledgeable about what we are putting into our bodies. But, it is not always clear to whom we should listen and who is providing unbiased information. This book is intended to be as objective and as current as possible by slicing through the mass of information available to you. At the same time, it aims to be comprehensive enough to give you a good sense of what you are getting before you eat or buy food.

Of course, as a nutritionist, people often ask me what they should eat. Since their ears are primed to receive only a sound-byte of truth, I often reply with this simple rule: If an item was in existence more than 100 years ago, it's probably safe. Otherwise, you may have to do some detective work to dissect your meal constituents. Since the advent of industrialization a bit more than 100 years ago, we have witnessed the proliferation of processed foods. Human-designed packaged food items cannot exist without their additive friends—the two go hand in hand. Over the years, we have gone from a sprinkling of salt to preserve and a bit of sugar to sweeten to an entire constellation of chemicals that pollute every bite. As you'll find out, many of these can have questionable effects on your health, while others may even be helpful.

The best rule of thumb is to keep your foods *simple*—whole, unprocessed foods in their natural state are ideal and highly recommended (see Table 1). These foods are what I like to call "naked"—sold without the dressing of plastic, metal, cardboard, or Styrofoam. Next are products with uncomplicated ingredient lists that contain actual food constituents rather than synthetic additives. Finally, if there are some "unpronounceables" in the list, ensure that they are minimal and not artificial anything—artificial colors, preservatives, flavors, or sweeteners.

Table 1. How Do Your Foods Measure Up?

Rating	Characteristics
Ideal	Not adulterated or processed, in "whole" form
	Freshly picked or collected
	Organically grown
	Additive-free
	Usually no package, no label
	Bought in "bulk" (in supermarket)
	Obtained from personal or neighborhood gardens, farms, farmers' markets, select supermarkets
	Examples: Fruits, eggs, vegetables, nuts, seeds, fresh meats, cereals, grains
Very Good	Minimally packaged
	Some organic ingredients
	Simple ingredients that are recognizable and pronounceable
	Few or no food additives
	Obtained in supermarkets
	Examples: Canned or dry legumes, packaged dried fruit, select snack bars, packaged trail mix, steel-cut oatmeal, salted nuts, tofu, cheeses

Rating	Characteristics
Above Average	Packaged
	Handful of ingredients (about 5 to 7)
	Ingredients mostly pronounceable
	Not excessively high in sugar, salt, or fat
	Food additives present
	Original forms eaten years ago have been replaced with a current version modified by chemicals and technology
	Obtained in supermarkets, convenience stores, delis
	Examples: High-fiber crackers, whole-grain breads, select ready-to-eat cereals, cheeses, low-fat yogurts, soups, select salad dressings
Fair	Packaged
	Long list of ingredients (usually 8 to 10)
	Majority of ingredients chemical in nature
	Ingredients not easily pronounceable, but somewhat recognizable
	Moderately high in sugar, fat, or salt
	Several additives mentioned
	May be labeled as "enriched" or "fortified" or other wordy claims—all subtle indications that the product has been severely human-manipulated rather than "nature-inspired"

Rating	Characteristics
	Obtained in supermarkets, bakeries, convenience stores, delis
	Examples: Cake mixes, prepackaged muffins, instant desserts, sauces, margarines, spreads, beverages, ketchup, breakfast bars
Think Twice Before Buying	Packaged
	Overwhelming list of ingredients (usually more than 10)
	Some ingredients may be questionable; they are long, complex, unpronounceable, and mention the adjectives *artificial* or *hydrogenated*
	High in sugar or fat
	Long list of food additives, or the majority of ingredients are food additives
	Sources of "anti-nutrition" in your diet, meaning they deplete your nutritional reserves
	Obtained in supermarkets, bakeries, convenience stores, delis, vending machines, fast-food restaurants, airports
	Examples: Soft drinks, candy bars, premade cakes, glazed donuts, toaster pastries, snack foods, gelatin desserts, spreads, frozen desserts, frozen entrees

Labeling Basics

To understand food additives, you need to understand some key aspects of the food label to help you put things in perspective. The ingredients on a food label are given in order of greatest quantity by weight. For example, on a label that reads "black beans, water, corn syrup, salt," black beans compose the largest amount of the weight of the food product, with salt the smallest. Now, you may be asking yourself, *Where are the "food additives" lurking?* In the case of black beans, corn syrup and salt would be classic, intentional food additives, since they add flavor. Water and salt may also be used as part of the processing and packaging, causing them to fall under the food-additive category as well.

Food additives can go beyond basics like water and salt and into the realm of chemically refined substances like artificial sweeteners and colorings. There is often a fine line between an additive and an ingredient. Several processed foods have become amalgams of what we may call additives—products like hard candy and marshmallows, which are both composed almost entirely of sweeteners, colorings, and flavorings. Many times, it may not be clear what you are really eating and what kinds of effects it may have on you if you consume it over a period of years. Some additives have been tested extensively by themselves, but often not in combination with the food matrix and other additives. And some have only been tested in animals and not humans.

It is not surprising that people often question whether food additives actually "subtract" from the nutritional quality of food. Certain additives may give us nutrition, others may be more neutral, and there are even those that deplete us of nutrients ("anti-nutrients") (see Table 2). You may find that some of the additives in this book cause more damage than good; others may be necessary. No doubt you'll also find a lot of gray in between.

Certain additives may give us nutrition, others may be more neutral, and there are even those that deplete us of nutrients. We might call these "anti-nutrients."

Table 2. The Additive Continuum

Additive Value	Description	Category	Example
Nutritious	Additives that impart some health benefit, usually due to their nutritional value or action in the body	Fiber, minerals, vitamins, natural antioxidants, probiotics	Beta-carotene, chlorophyll, vitamin E, lycopene, psyllium, inulin, bifidobacteria
Neutral	Additives that have essentially little or no impact on health	Acids, bases, salts, starches, phosphates	Citric acid, ammonium bicarbonate, calcium chloride, modified food starch
Depleting	Additives that take away from valuable body reserves	Artificial sweeteners, colorings, and flavorings; fat substitutes; partially hydrogenated oils; preservatives	Olestra, sucralose, FD&C Yellow No. 5, BHT, MSG, sulfites

Hot Topics

Here are some "hot topics" that relate to food additives that can help you evaluate the foods you buy and eat.

Organic foods: Food products labeled as "organic" indicate that some or all additives and/or ingredients used in the item were produced through organic farming practices. Organic ingredients are grown without chemicals like synthetic fertilizers, pesticides, insecticides, herbicides, antibiotics, and growth hormones. They are not genetically modified or irradiated. The land that these foods are grown on has to be free of chemicals for at least three years, and the farm is subject to inspection by a certifying agency.

Gluten-free foods: Our awareness about the gluten content of foods continues to expand. Gluten is a common protein food constituent and additive that should be avoided by individuals with celiac disease, a serious intestinal disorder that can be alleviated by avoiding gluten. Newer research suggests that a continuum of gluten intolerance may exist, meaning that one does not have to have celiac disease to be sensitive to gluten. Often, people believe that if a product is labeled as "wheat free," it is "gluten free"; however, this may not be accurate. In many "wheat-free" products like bread and crackers, another gluten-containing grain (usually a grain called "spelt") may be substituted in its place. Therefore, if you are gluten intolerant, it is best to read the ingredient label *very carefully*. Generally, products made from barley, rye, oats, wheat, or spelt (remember the acronym: BROWS) contain gluten. Of course, this list is not exhaustive. Relatives of these grains are also culprits that can trigger a response. There are several food additives that contain these grains as a starter source. For example, hydrolyzed wheat protein, an ingredient widely used in processed foods, contains gluten. Even modified food starch can potentially contain gluten if derived from wheat. Corn and rice are good substitutes for gluten-containing grains.

Genetically modified organisms (GMOs): GMO foods and food additives, which first appeared on the market in the 1990s, are those that have had their genetic material (DNA) altered through genetic engineering. Common genetically modified foods include those from soy (about 80 percent of U.S. crops), corn, cottonseed oil, tomato, and rapeseed (canola). Genetic engineering involves taking DNA from two different organisms, like a tomato plant and a cotton plant, and putting them together to form one DNA molecule. This practice is usually employed for specific genes and properties in an organism. For instance, GMOs have been used to help create plants that are more resistant to pests. GMOs are not allowed in the European Union, and there is some controversy as to whether they should be permitted in the United States. Concerns have been raised over the long-term effects of these organisms in the larger context of the ecosystem and also their long-term impact on human health. One potential health issue is the formation of new food allergens, toxins, and diseases.

Common genetically modified foods include those from soy (about 80 percent of U.S. crops), corn, cottonseed oil, tomato, and rapeseed (canola).

Bovine growth hormone: Recombinant bovine growth hormone (rBGH or rBST) has been the subject of much discussion since its commercial use began in 1993. This hormone is made naturally by cows and can be produced using special genetic engineering techniques ("recombinant DNA technology"). It is injected into cows so that they produce more milk. Certainly, rBGH-injected cows produce 11–16 percent more milk, but an extensive analysis of several published studies by researchers at the Atlantic Veterinary College at the University of Prince Edward Island in 2003 showed that cattle treated with rBGH are at high risk for mastitis (inflammation of the mammary gland), infertility, and becoming lame. Because these cows tend to become infected, they are treated with large doses of antibiotics. Of course, these antibiotics may show up in the milk. In addition to the risks to animals treated with rBGH, there is also concern for human safety. Since there have been no long-term studies on the effects of people drinking milk from cows treated with rBGH, there is no conclusive evidence either way. Unless your milk states that it does not contain hormones (is "bGH free") or is organic, chances are high that it does, since rBGH is used by thousands of dairy producers.

Fair trade products: Fair trade refers to an international social movement supported by a host of social, religious, environmental, and development groups that aims to reduce global poverty and promote sustainability by fostering opportunities for economically disadvantaged populations in rural communities. International trade organizations oversee the network of trade to ensure that it abides by certain principles like payment of a fair price for labor without discrimination by gender or race. Popular fair-trade products include coffee, cocoa, bananas, fruit, wine, cotton, sugar, tea, honey, and vanilla. You may see a symbol denoting that a given food is a fair-trade product, or you may see specific ingredients or additives listed in the ingredient list that specify they are fair-trade items. Common fair-trade additives are sugar, vanilla, honey, and cocoa.

Popular fair-trade products include coffee, cocoa, bananas, fruit, wine, cotton, sugar, tea, honey, and vanilla.

Beware the Not-So-Sweet Sugar Substitutes

Five artificial sweeteners (also known as synthetic sweeteners or sugar substitutes) have crept into many foods and beverages in the United States. They sit in little colored packages on restaurant tables and in large heavy-duty, resealable bags on grocery shelves so that we can bake with them. Many of them are now quite pronounceable because their long chemical descriptors have been converted into short, catchy names or names that sound like sugar so you won't know the difference (see Table 3).

People like these substitutes because they make foods taste intensely sweet without the burden of the calories that normally come with adding sugar. Sound too good to be true? Most likely it is. This gift of heavenly sweetness doesn't come without some hidden trade-offs. Although many of them are well tested in laboratory studies with cells, animals, and people, an underground of Web sites, blogs, and anecdotes have surfaced over the years claiming that they can have a variety of negative effects on health, often related to the brain (behavior) and nervous system (headaches, dizziness, nausea, hallucinations). It is not unreasonable to think that some individuals may be sensitive to their effects, depending on the foods that contain them and the quantities in which they are eaten.

What I have consistently observed with people is that excessive daily use of artificial sweeteners paves the way to overeating and cravings. Even though studies are out there on these sweeteners, there is likely some research left undone. Many of these artificial sweeteners have not been on the market long enough to see their long-term effects. Recently, two Purdue University scientists showed that, when laboratory rats are fed saccharin, they eat more and weigh more than rats that are fed glucose. The researchers suggested that artificial sweeteners may interfere with our physiological responses to food. In light of this study, it would be interesting to explore whether the increased use of artificial sweeteners in recent decades is linked to the obesity crisis.

One of the newest sugar substitutes, sucralose (Splenda®), is a sugar molecule with three chlorine atoms hanging onto it (see figure 1). Chlorine is a well-documented toxin. Therefore, it is not unreasonable to suspect that large amounts of chlorine, or even small amounts, coming into contact with the gut (often referred to as "the second brain") may trigger effects throughout the body. Indeed, anecdotal reports suggest that sucralose ingestion causes everything from red, itchy patches to bloating to headaches. Even though well-designed studies exist to show that sucralose is nontoxic, what hasn't been taken into account are individual physiologies and genetic material (DNA). Everyone is so different in body make-up that it is difficult to predict which sweeteners will affect a particular physiology. It is probable, however, that there will be some interaction.

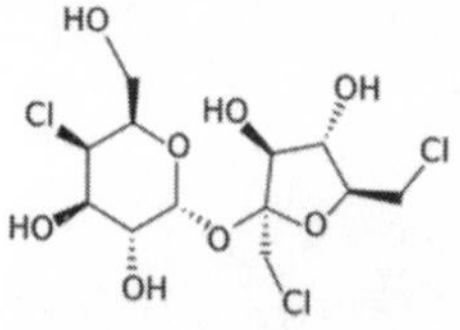

Figure 1. Sucralose molecule

Although there are mixed opinions on this issue, my personal recommendation is to keep artificial sweeteners out of the diet as much as possible. Not only because we don't know how our bodies will interact with them, but also, as the name suggests, because they are "artificial"—

meaning not natural. If you ingest an artificially inflated sense of sweetness all the time, think how difficult it will be to come back down to earthy, healthy, whole foods that have a fraction of that exaggerated sweetness. Make it easier on your taste buds by sticking to natural sweeteners.

If you ingest an artificially inflated sense of sweetness all the time, think how difficult it will be to come back down to earthy, healthy, whole foods that have a fraction of that exaggerated sweetness.

Table 3. Common Names of Artificial Sweeteners

Common Name(s)	Chemical Name(s)
Acesulfame K, Ace K, Sunett®, Sweet One®	Potassium 6-methyl-2,2-dioxo-oxathiazin-4-olate
Aspartame, NutraSweet®, Tropicana Slim®, Equal®, Canderel®	*N*-(L-α-Aspartyl)-L-phenylalanine, 1-methyl ester
Neotame	(3*R*)-3-(3,3-Dimethylbutylamino)-4-[[(1*R*)-2-methoxy-2-oxo-1-(phenylmethyl)ethyl]amino]-4-oxobutanoic acid

Common Name(s)	Chemical Name(s)
Splenda®, sucralose	1,6-Dichloro-1,6-dideoxy-ß-D-fructofuranosyl-4-chloro-4-deoxy-α-D-galactopyranoside
Sweet 'N Low®, saccharin	1,1-Dioxo-1,2-benzothiazol-3-one (note: Sweet 'N Low contains saccharin plus dextrose and cream of tartar)

Stay on the Bright End of the Rainbow

Why do people in the Mediterranean live longer and have a lower incidence of disease? Some people say it's because of what they eat. Their diet is full of fresh (non-additive laden) fruits, fish, vegetables, whole grains, legumes, and nuts. Individuals in these cultures drink red wine and use copious amounts of olive oil. Why is that food pattern healthy? One reason is that they are eating a palette of colors—reds, oranges, yellows, greens, purples, browns, tans, and whites. More and more research is surfacing that shows us the benefits of the thousands of colorful "phytochemicals" (*phyto*=plant) that exist in foods. These healthful, non-nutritive compounds in plants provide color and function to the plant and add to the health of the human body. Each color connects to a particular compound that serves a specific function in the body. For example, if you don't eat purple foods, you are probably missing out on anthocyanins, important brain protection compounds. Similarly, if you avoid green-colored foods, you may be lacking chlorophyll, a plant antioxidant that guards your cells from damage. Some of these phytochemicals, like lycopene (a red compound), are extracted from their plant sources and added to foods or dietary supplements to make them more nourishing and colorful (see Table 4).

Color catches our eye (it has been said that people "eat with their eyes"), and we associate certain colors with particular flavors or characteristics. For example, most people know that butter is yellow, but the reason butter is yellow is because of the addition of food colorings. Food colorings can be used by food manufacturers to enhance the coloring of a food and make it true to the color with which we associate it—like adding red dyes to meats to make them look more palatable rather than their natural brownish color, or making candy in bright rainbow colors to appeal to a larger group of consumers. Adding color results in consistent appearance in foods that may vary from one crop to the next due to changes in growing seasons and extremes in temperature, moisture, light, and air.

On the other end of the rainbow, opposite the pot of gold of healthy colorful compounds, we have the spectrum of artificial food colorings. This family of seven certified color additives (known by names that start with "FD&C," which stands for Foods, Drugs, and Cosmetics) differs from the naturally occurring plant compounds in that they are more concentrated and uniform and can therefore be added to foods in smaller quantities and provide consistent results without the flavors that are attached to natural colorings like beets. Despite these seemingly positive attributes for food applications, these food colorings have been criticized for causing a variety of negative effects in the body. Some individuals are sensitive to the effects of the FD&C-approved colorings and can develop allergic-type symptoms (for example, hives) when eating foods that contain them. There is some discussion as to whether certain colorings cause cancer in humans.

Table 4. Natural and Artificial Food Colorings

COLOR	RED
Foods	Meat, snack food coatings, gelatins, puddings, milks, cereals, cherries, biscuits, canned fruit, condiments, popcorn oil, candies, beverages, fruit fillings, salad dressings, cheeses
Natural Forms	Annatto extract, astaxanthin, beet powder, cochineal extract (carmine), lycopene, paprika extract
Health Effects	Annatto can cause allergic reactions in sensitive individuals; Astaxanthin is an antioxidant; Beet powder has no toxic effects when tested in high amounts in rats; Cochineal extract can cause allergic reactions in sensitive individuals; Lycopene is an antioxidant and possible anti-cancer agent; Paprika extract contains capsanthin, an antioxidant that may have health benefits (paprika also belongs to the nightshade family of plants and should be avoided by those who are sensitive).
Artificial Forms	FD&C Red No. 40 (Allura Red AC), FD&C Red No. 3 (Erythrosine)
Health Effects	Possible cancer risk; Ingestion may lead to behavioral abnormalities such as attention deficit disorder and hyperactivity; Possibility of allergic reactions. Rat study indicated that Red No. 3 may cause thyroid tumors.
COLOR	**ORANGE**
Foods	Cereals, baked goods, snack foods, confections, beverages, ice cream

Natural Forms	Beta-carotene, canthaxanthin, carrot oil, lutein, zeaxanthin
Health Effects	Beta-carotene is an antioxidant, converts in body to Vitamin A; Canthaxanthin is an antioxidant; Lutein and zeaxanthin are antioxidants that collect in eye tissue.
Artificial Froms	FD&C Yellow No. 6 (Sunset Yellow)
Health Effects	May promote allergic reactions, particularly in sensitive individuals with asthma and rhinitis. Possible cancer risk.
COLOR	**YELLOW**
Foods	Dairy products (cheese, ice cream), confections, salad dressings, fish, pickles, snack foods, cereals, soft drinks, juices
Natural Forms	Riboflavin (Vitamin B2), saffron, turmeric (curcumin)
Health Effects	Riboflavin aids in metabolism of nutrients, red blood cell formation, cell respiration; Saffron may be an anti-cancer agent, but high amounts (gram levels) may be toxic; Turmeric is an anti-inflammatory and an antioxidant, and may be anti-carcinogenic.
Artificial Forms	FD&C Yellow No. 5 (Tartrazine)
Health Effects	May promote asthma attacks, rash, hives, behavioral disturbances in sensitive individuals; Possible cancer risk.

Table 4. Natural and Artificial Food Colorings *(cont.)*

COLOR	GREEN
Foods	Baked goods, soups, frozen desserts, confections, sauces, beverages, puddings, ice cream, dairy products, vegetables
Natural Forms	Chlorophyll and chlorophyllin
Health Effects	May act as antioxidants.
Artificial Forms	FD&C Green No. 3 (Fast Green FCF)
Health Effects	Causes caner when injected into animals.
COLOR	**BLUE**
Foods	Beverages, dairy products, jellies, confections, icings, syrups, extracts, snack foods, ice cream
Natural Forms	None
Health Effects	None
Artificial Forms	FD&C Blue No. 1 (Brilliant Blue FCF), FD&C Blue No. 2 (Indigotine)
Health Effects	May cause allergic reactions in sensitive individuals.
COLOR	**PURPLE**
Foods	Grape and other fruit juices, vegetable juice
Natural Forms	Grape color extract (anthocyanin)
Health Effects	Anthocyanins, the water-soluble blue pigment in grapes and blueberries, are antioxidants that may be important in eye health, immunity, and reducing risk of heart disease.

Artificial Forms	None
Health Effects	None
COLOR	BROWN
Foods	Beer, bread, buns, chocolate, cookies, coatings, desserts, gravy, pancakes, sauces, soft drinks (colas), alcoholic beverages
Natural Forms	Caramel color
Health Effects	Possible cancer-causing agent.
Artificial Forms	None
Health Effects	None
COLOR	BLACK
Foods	Black olives
Natural Forms	Ferrous gluconate
Health Effects	Provides source of iron.
Aritificial Forms	None
Health Effects	None

Favor Safe Flavorings

Flavoring agents belong to a broad category of food additives that contains about 2,000 different flavorings, of which a majority (about 1,500) are synthetic. Natural flavorings like garlic, ginger, orange oil, and peppermint are generally safe, but are rarely used instead of artificial flavorings due to cost. Although artificial flavorings are probably less toxic than artificial food colorings, they tend to be more widespread in foods, including soft drinks, ice cream, baked goods, puddings, gelatins, sauces, dressings, and candy. If a food contains a natural or artificial flavoring, the package will tell you so, but will typically provide no details on the names of the flavorings used. Again, the best rule of thumb is to avoid "artificial" ingredients altogether.

Keeping Your Food Fresh

Of course, making food convenient means that is has to be able to survive without spoiling. In their raw form, foods are vulnerable to attack by bacteria, fungi, and even oxygen, so they need protection if they are going to last.

Antioxidants like BHA, BHT, and sodium benzoate help to ward off the negative effects of oxygen. You'll find them in products like fats and oils to keep them from going rancid. Although these preservatives may keep your food fresh, they may also give you headaches, difficulty breathing, hives, nausea, and digestive complaints. Some synthetic antioxidants may also have questionable effects on cancer development or progression. In addition to unknown effects on cancer, it is thought that these substances are highly allergenic and can provoke responses like difficulty breathing in people who are sensitive to them, such as asthmatics.

Other categories of preservatives that may be less dangerous than antioxidants are bacteria and mold inhibitors like calcium propionate and sorbic acid. These agents are often added to foods prone to spoiling or becoming moldy, like breads, baked goods, and cheeses. Although they need to be considered on an individual basis, most are considered safe. Sulfites and nitrites are antimicrobials that are under intense scrutiny because they are allergenic additives and, in the case of nitrites, cancer causing.

The Perils of Silent Additives

Some additives are incorporated into foods deliberately. Others—such as toxic chemical pollutants in water and air, heavy metals in the fish supply, and pesticides on conventionally grown foods—make their way into our food in less obvious ways. Much attention has been given to the subtle, silent, potentially harmful additives that appear in foods without being labeled or measured. One example of this is food packaging. Plastic packages—including plastic wraps, water bottles, and baby bottles—are among the worst offenders. Aside from the fact that plastics are petroleum based (and thus, not a sustainable resource), they create excess waste and contain chemicals that leach into foods and beverages. Ones to watch for are polycarbonate, polyvinyl chloride, and polystyrene plastics. They contain chemicals like bisphenol A, which disrupts hormones and can stimulate certain cancers.

Here are some quick tips to avoiding the dangers present in some food packaging:

1. Do not heat food in plastic containers. Place in a glass dish or on a plate.

2. Minimize your use of cling wraps. Package foods in glass containers.
3. Reduce the amount of foods you eat from cans. Many cans are lined with bisphenol A.
4. Do not drink out of plastic bottles. Stainless steel or glass is a better alternative.

Another insidious food additive is the heavy metal methylmercury, which appears in the water supply due to a variety of industrial processes, like power plants that burn coal and automobile scrap recycling. This toxic compound gradually accumulates in algae and travels up the food chain into the largest fish (see Table 5). Repeated ingestion of large, contaminated fish by people causes developmental problems in children and cardiovascular disease in adults. Consumption of fish low in methylmercury is advised by health authorities. Pregnant women, women planning to become pregnant, lactating women, and young children are advised by the Environmental Protection Agency and FDA to limit fish intake to low-mercury choices no more than twice a week (or a total of twelve ounces per week).

Table 5. Incidence of Methylmercury in Fish

High-Methyl-mercury Fish		Low-Methyl-mercury Fish	
Dangerously High	**Considerably High**	**Low**	**Low (cont.)**
Mackerel (King) Marlin* Orange Roughy* Shark* Swordfish* Tilefish* Tuna (Bigeye, Ahi)*	Bluefish Grouper* Mackerel (Spanish, Gulf) Sea Bass (Chilean)* Tuna (Canned Albacore) Tuna (Yellowfin)*	Anchovies Butterfish Catfish Clam Crab (Domestic) Crawfish/Crayfish Croaker (Atlantic) Flounder* Haddock (Atlantic)* Hake Herring Mackerel (N. Atlantic, Chub) Mullet	Oyster Perch (Ocean) Pollock Salmon (Canned) Salmon (Fresh) Sardine Scallop* Shrimp* Sole (Pacific) Squid (Calamari) Trout (Freshwater) Whitefish Whiting

Source: Natural Resources Defense Council *nrdc.org/health/effects/mercury/guide.asp*

* Indicates shortage due to overfishing

Top Twelve Additives to Avoid in an Ideal World

Here is a list that can help you avoid the worst offenders of food additives.

1. **Salt** (sodium chloride). Eating lots of processed foods means a greater chance of eating large amounts of salt. Too much salt impacts your hydration status and can ultimately affect blood pressure. Some individuals are more sensitive to these effects than others.
2. **Sugar** (comes in many forms). Sugars are pervasive in the food supply and have been compared to working like a "drug" in that they can be addictive. Numerous health consequences (dental caries, obesity, diabetes) can result from overconsumption.
3. **Trans fats** (partially hydrogenated oils). These food-industry-created fats can be considered "artificial," because they are made through the chemical process of hydrogenation. They have deleterious effects on your blood fats (like decreasing your "good" cholesterol and increasing your "bad"

cholesterol) and are not perceived as being healthy for your heart.

4. **Monosodium glutamate** (MSG). MSG has the potential to provoke serious bodily reactions like headaches, anxiety, fast heart rate, chest tightness, and tingling muscles.

5. **Artificial anything** (colorings, flavorings, sweeteners). "Artificial" denotes questionable effects in the body, since these are not compounds found in nature. All three categories mentioned have had varying degrees of negative effects associated with them.

6. **Nitrates and nitrites**. Preservatives commonly found in preserved meats that may further react in the body to become cancer agents.

7. **Sulfites**. Preservatives found in fruits (especially grapes and wines, dried fruits) that may cause allergic reactions like respiratory difficulty, headache, nausea, and digestive complaints.

8. **BHT/BHA.** Preservatives in products like soups, cereals, oils, and crackers may cause allergic reactions and neuro-toxic effects, including hyperactivity.
9. **Fat substitutes.** Non-absorbable, synthetic fat substitutes in snack foods like potato chips can lead to severe digestive complaints.
10. **Potassium bromate.** This compound, which is added to improve the structure of flour within bread-type products, has been banned in several countries (not in the United States) because it causes cancer in animals.
11. **Gluten.** Gluten is added to bread products to make them rise better. It also occurs naturally in grains. Due to improved testing methods and greater awareness, people are finding they can be "gluten intolerant" without having celiac disease. Various reasons for this rise may include changing strains of wheat through genetic modification, impaired immunity, or simply the sheer number of products that contain it and the frequency with which they are eaten—or a combination of any of these factors.

12. **White flour.** White flour has typically been refined and chemically bleached with peroxides or chlorine to the point where it needs to be enriched or have synthetic nutrients added back to it. The problem is that it doesn't get close to resembling its natural state—full of vitamins, minerals, and fiber. Foods containing predominantly white flour may raise blood sugar and make your body work harder to metabolize it due to its high glycemic index.

Put Your Learning to the Test

This list of additives you should avoid clearly indicates that there are some ingredients that do more harm than good. It is important to sift through the rows of ingredients in the list on a package label to be sure that you are minimizing your intake of these substances. Worse yet, many of these additives can be combined into one product. Remember that, for the most part, food-additive safety standards do not take into account effects that may arise from combining additives into a matrix. Often, if we are lucky, we only know how they work in isolation.

With all that in mind, consider the following ingredients found on an actual label (brand withheld) of white sourdough bread:

> **Enriched White Flour** (**Malted Barley Flour, Potassium Bromate**, Niacin, Iron, Thiamine, Riboflavin), **White Sugar**, Soybean Oil (Citric Acid), Whey Solids, less than 1% Calcium Stearoyl Lactylate, **Corn Syrup Solids**, Soy Protein Isolate, **Partially Hydrogenated Oils (Palm Kernel, Soybean & Cotton Seed**), Soy Lecithin, Calcium & Sodium Caseinate, Mono- & Di-glycerides, Sodium Acid Pyrophosphate, **Sodium Bisulfite**, **BHT**, Vitamin C (Ascorbic Acid), Dipotassium Phosphate, **Artificial Flavor**, Yeast, **Salt**, Water

How many of the forbidden additives do you see? The boldfaced type shows that there are over ten ingredients that are in the "no-no" category. Bread happens to be one of those products loaded with heavy hitters. Of course, the primary ingredient is white flour, a known "forbidden" substance because it's been bleached and stripped of nutrients. Also, we know it contains gluten from the barley.

Potassium bromate, a known carcinogen banned from a number of countries, was added to the flour to help it make a firm, yet cushy bread. Note that there is not only one source of sugar, but two: "white sugar" (they make it sound even more dangerous by specifying "white") and "corn syrup solids" (did you catch this one?). The bread manufacturer wanted to be sure we got our daily sampler of trans fat by giving us a selection of three different partially hydrogenated oils. And, of course—the best for last—we get to savor sulfites, BHT, artificial flavor, and salt. Now I know where my mom got the phrase, "The whiter the bread, the quicker you're dead!"

With foods like these filling the supermarket aisles, you have to be fully conscious and aware each time you make a food purchase. Every selection you make can have great implications in the long run!

Learning the Lingo

Being familiar with the vocabulary of food additives can help you navigate the grocery store shelves more easily. Here are some categories of food additives to look for.

Acid: Fulfills a multitude of functions—intensifies flavor, provides sour taste, controls microorganism growth, coagulates proteins (needed for cheese formation), reduces rancidity or breakdown of the product due to oxygen exposure. Examples: citric acid, lactic acid.

Alkali: Reduces acidity of a food to enhance flavor, change functional properties, and prevent microorganism growth. Examples: ammonium bicarbonate, sodium bicarbonate.

Anti-caking agent: Prevents particles, powders, or granular ingredients from clumping and sticking together. Example: aluminum sodium salt.

Anti-foaming agent: Prevents unwanted foaming in foods during processing. Example: polydimethylsiloxane.

Antimicrobial: Prevents the growth of harmful microorganisms. Example: potassium metabisulfite.

Antioxidant: Increases shelf life of foods by protecting them from degradation through exposure to oxygen; may be natural or artificial in origin; may have health benefits. Examples: Vitamin E (tocopherols), BHT.

Artificial sweetener: Often referred to as "synthetic" or "non-nutritive" sweeteners. Sweetens foods intensely (sometimes hundreds or thousands times as sweet as white sugar); often used for diabetic food products because it does not impact blood sugar levels. Many do not contain calories. Side effects related to ingestion include headaches, mood swings, blurred vision, weight gain, skin rashes, and behavioral changes. Examples: sucralose (Splenda®), aspartame (NutraSweet®).

Buffer: Controls pH (acidity or alkalinity) within a product. Example: potassium citrate.

Bulking agent: Adds mass to a food without significantly changing its nutritional qualities. Example: carboxymethylcellulose.

Chelating agent: Binds metals to prevent them from reacting with other food ingredients like fats. Example: EDTA.

Color stabilizer: Retains or intensifies the natural color and brightness of a food item. Example: calcium phosphate.

Dough conditioner: Assists in the appearance or function of baked products. Examples: calcium stearoyl lactylate, mono- and diglycerides.

Emulsifier: Allows two or more immiscible (non-mixing) substances (such as fats and water) to come together in a medium ("emulsion"). Example: lecithin.

Fat: Macronutrient used for energy (9 calories per gram) and for key functions in the body. Has a slippery, creamy feel in the mouth; comes in solid and liquid forms. May be naturally-occurring or synthesized. Example: palmitic acid, partially hydrogenated vegetable oil.

Fat substitute: Chemically synthesized compound made to mimic the sensory properties of fat (creamy, smooth, slippery) without the same amount of calories as fat. Examples: Salatrim®, olestra (Olean®).

Fiber: A non-digestible carbohydrate that can be "soluble" or "insoluble" in water, giving it beneficial health properties such as slowing the release of glucose into the blood stream and improving the motility of the gastrointestinal tract. Examples: inulin, psyllium.

Firming agent: Keeps texture of fruits and vegetables firm. Example: tetrasodium phosphate.

Flavoring agent: Gives flavor to a product that may or may not have been lost in processing. May be natural or artificially synthesized. Example: calcium chloride.

Flavor, artificial: Imparts a specific aroma or taste to a food that is not naturally present; synthetically derived. Example: isoamyl acetate.

Flavor, natural: Imparts a specific aroma or taste to a food; from natural, non-adulterated sources. Example: vanillin.

Flavor enhancer: Intensifies the inherent flavor of a food; from natural or chemically derived sources. Example: hydrolyzed vegetable protein.

Food coloring: Adds color to a food depleted of its natural color due to processing or to enhance the presentation of food. May be naturally obtained or synthetically derived. In the U.S., FD&C numbers (indicating that they can be used in "Food, Drug & Cosmetics") are assigned to individual synthetic colorings. Several synthetic colorings have been thought to be toxic and associated with cancer, attention deficit disorders, and general allergic reactions. Examples: FD&C Red No. 40, caramel color.

Gelling agent: Provides texture in a food by assisting in gel formation. Select stabilizers and thickeners can be considered gelling agents. Example: gelatin.

Glazing agent: Coats a food to protect it or give it a glossy appearance. Example: beeswax.

Humectant: Provides or helps retain moisture in a food. Example: corn syrup.

Leavening agent: Increases the volume in foods through its ability to manufacture carbon dioxide gas. Example: ammonium bicarbonate.

Nutrient: May be a "macronutrient" (protein, carbohydrate, or fat) or a "micronutrient" (vitamin, mineral) added to a food through the process of enrichment (replacing nutritional value lost in food processing) or fortification (enhancing nutritional value over and above what would naturally be found in the food). Examples: Vitamin A, fat.

Preservative: Increases shelf life of food by reducing its susceptibility to spoilage by microorganisms. Example: calcium propionate.

Stabilizer: Provides foods with a stronger texture by ensuring a uniform dispersion of immiscible (non-mixing) substances. Example: pectin.

Sweetener: Imparts a sweet taste to foods. May include artificial and natural sweeteners (including sugar alcohols and stevia). Example: corn syrup.

Texturizer: Assists a food in achieving desired consistency or texture. Example: casein.

Thickener: Increases viscosity without interfering with the food's other properties. Example: alginate made from seaweed.

Whipping agent: Used to increase and hold volume in foods. Example: sodium stearoyl lactylate.

An A-Z List of Food Additives

Following is an alphabetical list of the most common food additives you will find in products on your grocery shelves. I have rated them based on current science and regulations; they could change based on new findings. The following scale rates their impact on your health:

A+ = Safe to eat; may be nutritious

A = Safe to eat

B = Most likely safe, but cut back

C = Reasonably safe, but limit quantities

D = Safety questionable, try to avoid

F = Do not eat foods with this additive

Acacia gum. See Gums

Ace K. See Acesulfame-potassium

Acesulfame K. See Acesulfame-potassium

Acesulfame-potassium *(Acesulfame K, Ace K, Sunett®, Sweet One®, potassium 6-methyl-2,2-dioxo-oxathiazin-4-olate)*. Artificial sweetener. White, crystalline sweetener discovered in 1967, used in foods in the United States since 1988. 130–200 times sweeter than sugar; often blended with other artificial sweeteners to give a more true sugar taste. Heat stable and contributes no calories. According to FDA guidelines, it is a general-purpose sweetener to be added to all foods except meats. Found in thousands of foods, typically in soft drinks and other beverages, instant coffee and tea, gelatin and pudding desserts, syrups, baked goods, chewing gum. Acceptable daily intake set at 15 milligrams per kilogram body weight. Limited animal studies from more than two decades ago indicate it may cause cancer, although there is no definitive evidence to suggest that it is a carcinogen in humans. The Center for Science in the Public Interest (CSPI) has criticized the FDA for their lack of long-term animal studies using higher levels of the sweetener. CPSI has a Web site dedicated to quotes from cancer experts on its testing: *www.cspinet.org/reports/asekquot.html*. Rating: F

Acetic acid. Acid, flavor enhancer, preservative. Found naturally in plant and animal tissues as a product of carbohydrate fermentation. Added to a variety of products including baked goods, cheese, condiments, dairy products, gravies, mayonnaise, meats, oils, salad dressings, and sauces. Can be used as a pickling agent. Safe to consume when diluted and in small amounts such as those found in foods. If ingested in its pure form can cause severe damage (bleeding, ulcers) in the intestines. Rating: A

Agar *(agar-agar)*. Bulking agent, emulsifier, fiber, stabilizer, thickener. Mucilagenous substance from various seaweed sources used to thicken and stabilize desserts, soups, baked goods, frostings, and canned jellied meats. Used extensively in Asian foods and medicinally as a treatment for constipation. May have a laxative effect. Since it swells with water, may promote a feeling of fullness when eaten. May cause allergic reactions in sensitive individuals. Avoid if allergic. Rating: A+

Algin. See Alginate

Alginate *(alginic acid, algin, sodium alginate, pacific kelp)*. Bulking agent, emulsifier, fiber, stabilizer, thickener. Brown seaweed-derived ingredient that can stabilize foam and act as a thickener in products like jellies, salad dressings, beverages, custards, ice cream, soups, and cheese. Sodium alginate is the sodium salt form. Theoretically, due to its ability to trap dietary cholesterol in its gel-like structure, it may have cholesterol-lowering effects. Limited studies suggest it may create fullness or satiety, although this concept needs further testing. May cause allergic reactions in sensitive individuals. Avoid if allergic. Rating: A+

Alginic acid. See Alginate

Alpha tocopherol. See Vitamin E

Aluminum ammonium sulfate. Buffer. Odorless crystals with astringent taste used to purify drinking water and to manufacture baking powder. Two known cases of human poisoning when high amounts (30 grams) were eaten. Excessive amounts may cause digestive upset and nausea. Contains small amount of aluminum—it is unknown whether there is a causal association between aluminum ingestion and Alzheimer's disease. Rating: B

Aluminum calcium silicate. Anti-caking agent. Used in table salt (at 2 percent) and in vanilla powder. Contains a small amount of aluminum—it is unknown whether there is a causal association between aluminum ingestion and Alzheimer's disease. Rating: B

Ammonium bicarbonate *(bicarbonate of ammonia, ammonium hydrogen carbonate, hartshorn)*. Alkali, leavening agent. An alkali used in making baked goods, especially before baking soda was invented. Now sometimes used in conjunction with baking soda. Added to pesticides. Rating: A

Ammonium carrageenan. See Carrageenan

Ammonium chloride *(Sal Ammoniac, salmiac)*. Dough conditioner, flavor enhancer, leavening agent. Clear, white salt made by reacting sodium chloride (salt) with an ammonium salt. Used in baked goods, condiments, dairy products, margarine, dried and processed vegetables. Found in European candies. Higher amounts than those typically used in foods (0.5 to 1 gram) can cause nausea and vomiting. Rating: B

Ammonium hydrogen carbonate. See Ammonium bicarbonate

Ammonium phosphate. See Phosphates

Annatto extract. Food coloring, flavoring agent. Red food coloring derived from the tropical achiote tree. Imparts sweet peppery flavor. Used in dairy products (butter, cheeses), rice, smoked fish, dessert powders. Has potential to cause allergic reactions in sensitive individuals. Avoid if allergic. Rating: A

Anthocyanins. See Grape color extract

Arabic gum. See Gums

Artificial colorings *(FD&C Blue No. 1, FD&C Blue No. 2, FD&C Green No. 3, FD&C Red No. 3, FD&C Red No. 40, FD&C Yellow No. 5, FD&C Yellow No. 6, Orange B, Citrus Red No. 2).* Food coloring. Added to food to change its color. Usually found in low-nutrition foods; however, may also be added to "natural" foods like salmon to provide a more consistent tone in case of natural color variability. Recent studies suggest that artificial colorings cause hyperactivity and/or attention deficit disorder (ADD) in children. Some of these chemicals have led to formation of tumors in animals, but no proof exists that they do the same in humans. Hives and asthma have been reported in a small number of individuals who are particularly sensitive to FD&C Yellow No. 5. Allergic reactions are commonly associated with artificial colorings.

Researchers at the National College of Technology in Japan tested the toxicity of thirty-nine currently used food additives in eight mouse organs. They reported that dyes were most toxic, causing DNA damage in the stomach, colon, urinary bladder, and gut. Damage to the colon was with low doses of the dyes, in amounts comparable to the guidelines for acceptable

intake. There are nine certified colorings approved for used in the United States by the FDA. Seven are permitted for use in foods: FD&C Blue No. 1 (Brilliant Blue FCF), FD&C Blue No. 2 (Indigotine), FD&C Green No. 3 (Fast Green FCF), FD&C Red No. 3 (Erythrosine), FD&C Red No. 40 (Allura Red AC), FD&C Yellow No. 5 (Tartrazine), FD&C Yellow No. 6 (Sunset Yellow)
Rating: F

Ascorbate. See Vitamin C

Ascorbic acid. See Vitamin C

Ascorbyl palmitate. See Vitamin C

Aspartame *(NutraSweet®, Tropicana Slim, Equal®, Canderel, aspartyl-phenylalanine-1-methyl ester).* Artificial sweetener. Found in thousands of consumer food products. Commonly found in soft drinks, in individual packets as a condiment, or even in chewable vitamins. Not suitable for baked products because it breaks down in heat. Composed of methanol (10 percent) and two amino acids, L-aspartic acid (40 percent) and phenylalanine (50 percent). Therefore, individuals with the inherited metabolic disorder that prevents them from metabolizing the amino acid phenylalanine (called phenylketonuria or PKU) must avoid this sweetener.

Methanol breaks down in the body to a number of toxic metabolites such as formaldehyde. Formaldehyde production may be linked to incidence of migraines in aspartame users.

Animal studies have indicated that aspartame may cause negative health effects such as cancer. People have reported that it causes headaches, hallucinations, seizures, insomnia, and dizziness. Researchers Huff and LaDou from the National Institute of Environmental Health Sciences pointed out in 2007 that "the U.S. FDA should reevaluate its position on aspartame as being safe under all conditions."

Artificial sweeteners like aspartame are often used by Type 2 diabetics; however, Canadian researchers from Université Laval questioned the safety of use in this population due to their findings that a breakfast that contains aspartame led to the same rise in blood glucose and insulin as did a breakfast containing table sugar. This area of research needs further investigation. Rating: F

Astaxanthin. Food coloring, nutrient. Red pigment ("carotenoid") found naturally in algae, yeast, and fish (for example, salmon, krill) that can be used to color animal and fish foods. Used as fish feed and found in dietary supplements. Potent antioxidant, used throughout the body, especially in the central nervous system. May cause allergic reactions in individuals sensitive to fish or algae. Avoid if allergic. Rating: A+

Baking soda *(bicarbonate of soda, sodium bicarbonate, sodium hydrogen carbonate)*. Anti-caking, buffer, leavening agent, stabilizer. Fine, white, alkaline powder that combines with acidic ingredients or additives (lemon juice, cream of tartar, phosphates) to produce carbon dioxide gas, causing a food product to rise. Added to "self-rising" products like self-rising flour or self-rising corn meal, and incorporated into sweet baked goods (pastries, pies, cakes), breads, beverages, vegetable-based products, and cocoa products. Contains sodium. Limit if you are sodium sensitive. Rating: A

Beeswax. Flavoring agent, glazing agent. Honeybees secrete this waxy substance as part of honeycombs. Yellow beeswax is made commercially by removing honey from honeycomb, melting the comb, and refining the wax by melting and adding an acid or alkali to remove impurities. White beeswax involves bleaching the final product with peroxides or sunlight. Can be found in chewing gum and candies. Long history of safe use. Some individuals who may be sensitive to bee-derived products should avoid. Avoid if allergic. Rating: A

Beet powder. Food coloring. Dark red powder made from beets used to color candies, yogurt, ice cream, salad dressings, frostings, dessert mixes, meat substitutes, drink mixes, gravy mixes, and soft drinks. No toxic effects when tested in high amounts in rats. Rating: A

Benefat®. See Salatrim

Benzoic acid. See Sodium benzoate

Beta-carotene *(Vitamin A precursor).* Antioxidant, food coloring, nutrient. Orange pigment ("carotenoid") that occurs naturally in fruits and vegetables (for example, carrots). It can also be chemically synthesized. Often added to foods like margarine, shortening, and beverages to provide color. High amounts, more likely in supplemental form rather than foods, are not advocated for smokers. Once ingested, it can convert in the body to Vitamin A. Rating: A+

Beta-sitosterol. See Phytosterols/phytostanols

BHA. See Butylated hydroxyanisole

BHT. See Butylated hydroxytoluene

Bicarbonate of ammonium. See Ammonium bicarbonate

Bicarbonate of soda. See Baking soda

Brown sugar. See Sugar

Butylated hydroxyanisole *(BHA).* Antioxidant. Functions to protect fats from rancidity. Widely used in fat-containing products like meats (sausage, lunch meats), butter, lard, cereals, and baked goods. May have estrogen-like effects. A report from the National Institute of Health states that BHA is "reasonably anticipated to be a human carcinogen" since studies have demonstrated it causes cancer in rats, mice, and hamsters. There is, however, no scientific evidence that it causes cancer in humans. Rating: F

Butylated hydroxytoluene *(BHT).* Antioxidant. Functions to protect fats from rancidity; unknown whether it causes cancer due to mixed findings from animal studies. Acute, high doses (0.5 to 1.0 grams per kilogram—much higher than levels found in foods) have led to kidney and liver damage in male rats. Rats fed BHT at lower doses over a longer period of time developed enlarged livers and reduced liver enzyme activity. Has been linked to DNA damage in mouse gut. Has also been shown to prevent cancer in some experimental models. Rating: F

Caffeine. Flavoring agent. Naturally occurring substance in many plants and found in foods/drinks like coffee, cocoa, and tea. Added to cola-like beverages and "energy" drinks.

Stimulant effects, mildly addictive. May cause heart palpitations and insomnia in sensitive individuals. Avoid in pregnancy, since caffeine crosses the placenta. Avoid if sensitive or pregnant. Rating: C

Calcium ascorbate. See Vitamin C

Calcium bromate. Dough conditioner. Used in baked products like bread, rolls, and buns. Contains bromate, which may cause allergic reactions in sensitive individuals. Rating: F

Calcium carrageenan. See Carrageenan

Calcium caseinate. See Casein

Calcium chloride. Firming agent, flavoring agent. Keeps fruit firm. Used in sliced fruits, jellies, pie fillings. Found in bottled waters as an electrolyte. Its salty taste enables it to be used in canned vegetables and pickles without increasing sodium content. Also used in beer brewing. Rating: A

Calcium dihydrogen phosphate. See Monocalcium phosphate, Phosphates

Calcium disodium EDTA. See EDTA

Calcium gluconate *(calcium di-gluconate)*. Firming agent, nutrient, stabilizer, thickener. Calcium salt of gluconic acid (see

Gluconic acid). Added to dairy-based products, gelatins and puddings, frozen desserts, fruit preserves, bulk sugar substitutes, fermented soy products. Contains a small amount of calcium. Rating: A+

Calcium pantothenate. See Vitamin B5

Calcium phosphate. See Phosphates

Calcium or **Sodium propionate** *(propionic acid)*. Preservative. White or colorless crystalline solid that prevents bacteria and mold growth on products like bread, rolls, dairy products, processed sweet baked goods; also used to prevent fungal growth on growing produce. Unlike other preservatives, does not need an acidic environment to work. Can be found naturally (small amounts) in foods like cheese. Propionic acid is produced in the human body through metabolic processes. The calcium form of propionate is preferred from a functional perspective, since the alpha-amylase enzyme needs calcium to make the starch available to the yeast, allowing for better bread structure. Use of this additive in all forms is relatively widespread. There is debate about whether this additive is safe. Researchers have tested children's reactions to calcium propionate in bread against bread without calcium propionate. They found irritability, restlessness, inattention, and sleep disturbance in some children and advised minimizing concentrations added to processed foods. Sodium-sensitive individuals should limit or reduce their intake of sodium propionate. Rating: C

Calcium sorbate. See Sorbic acid

Calcium or **Sodium stearoyl lactylate** *(sodium stearoyl fumarate)*. Dough conditioner, emulsifier, whipping agent. Slightly sweet white powder made from the combination of lactic acid and the fatty acid, stearic acid, followed by treating it with either calcium hydroxide or sodium hydroxide to make the calcium or sodium salt, respectively. When fumaric acid (see Fumaric acid) is used in place of lactic acid, the final result is called sodium stearoyl fumarate. All forms of this additive toughen bread dough so that it can be processed with machinery. They create increased bread volume by making the gluten structure stronger and can assist as a whipping agent in egg and dairy products. Since this additive contains a fat, high amounts fed to rats caused fat to build up in the body. This effect was reversed by changing their diets. Although somewhat rare, lactose-intolerant persons may be sensitive to the lactylate forms, since lactic acid (made from fermenting lactose) is a starting ingredient. Avoid if lactose-intolerant;

sodium-sensitive individuals should limit the sodium form of this additive. Rating: A

Calcium sulfate. Bulking agent, emulsifier, stabilizer, thickener. White powder used in a variety of functions in dairy, egg, and meat products, frozen desserts, vegetables, confections, pasta, noodles, cereals, condiments, soups, sauces, and tofu. Found to be nontoxic in animal studies. Rating: A

Campesterol. See Phytosterols/phytostanols

Cane sugar. See Sugar

Canthaxanthin. Antioxidant, food coloring, nutrient. Orange-red pigment ("carotenoid") found in crustaceans, fish, and eggs. Primarily used as feed additive for animals to produce more intensely colored flesh and egg yolks. Less commonly added to fruit spreads, candies, syrups, beverages. May also be found in dietary supplements containing "mixed carotenoids." Levels found added to foods do not seem to result in intake that exceeds the Acceptable Daily Intake (ADI) of up to 0.03 milligrams per kilogram body weight. The amounts found in foods may be too insignificant for health effects. However, they may work in ways similar to other antioxidant carotenoids like beta-carotene (see Beta-carotene). Rating: A+

Capsanthin. See Paprika extract

Caramel color. Food coloring. Brown-colored substance made by heating sugar of any type (for example, corn syrup). Can be processed with ammonia and sulfur to intensify color. Used to intensify brown color in foods like beer, bread, buns, chocolate, cookies, coatings, desserts, gravy, pancakes, sauces, soft drinks (especially colas), and alcoholic beverages. There exists debate about its carcinogenicity. For caramel color without ammonia (types I and II), there is no limit on intake; however, for caramel color with ammonia (types III and IV), the acceptable daily intake is 0–200 milligrams per kilogram body weight. Researchers at the TNO Research Institute in the Netherlands demonstrated lowered immune function in rats fed caramel color III, especially in those with low levels of dietary vitamin B6. However, no changes in immune function of elderly men with low vitamin B6 status was noted when they were given this additive at 200 milligrams per kilogram body weight for seven days. Avoid if sensitive to corn. Rating: D

Carboxymethylcellulose *(Sodium carboxymethylcellulose, cellulose gum, CMC)*. Bulking agent, emulsifier, fiber, stabilizer, thickener. Odorless, white to yellow, water-soluble plant fiber (cellulose) derivative reacted with an acid. Sodium carboxymethylcellulose is the sodium salt of carboxymethylcellulose. Added to a variety of foods like ice cream, dressings, cheeses, icings, toppings, and gelatinous desserts. Also used as a binder (excipient) in dietary supplements. Considered a fiber source, used as a laxative in over-the-counter preparations. Sodium-sensitive individuals should note sodium source coming from sodium carboxymethylcellulose. Sodium-sensitive individuals should limit or reduce intake of sodium carboxymethylcellulose. Rating: A

Carmine. See Cochineal extract

Carnauba wax. Anti-caking agent, bulking agent, glazing agent. Wax obtained from Brazilian carnauba palm. Commercial grades contain saturated fatty acids and alcohols. Found in baked goods, baking mixes, chewing gum, fresh fruits, fruit juices, gravies, sauces, soft candy. Studies in animals at relatively high levels revealed no significant toxicity. Acceptable daily intake set at 0–7 milligrams per kilogram body weight. Rating: A

Carrageenan *(ammonium carrageenan, calcium carrageenan, potassium carrageenan, sodium carrageenan)*. Stabilizer, thickener. Long, non-digestible carbohydrates extracted from red seaweed (Irish moss, Chondrus crispus). May be used in ammonium, calcium, potassium, or sodium salt form. Small amounts of this seaweed-derived ingredient are used to stabilize and thicken processed foods like milk, ice cream, custards, dressings, and jellies. In Europe, not advocated for use in infant formulas due to unknown reactions with infant immature gut. When carrageenan is degraded with high heat and acid (called poligeenan) and fed to animals in large amounts, it has caused gastrointestinal ulcers and cancer. At the FAO/WHO Expert Committee on Food Additives meeting in June 2007, it was concluded that the inclusion of carrageenan in food products may need to be reevaluated. Rating: B

Carrot oil. Food coloring. Orange, oily extract from carrots that can be incorporated into sauces, salad dressings, meat seasonings, pasta, margarine. Contains carotenoids like beta-carotene, which may have health-promoting effects. Rating: A+

Casein *(calcium caseinate, potassium caseinate, sodium caseinate)*. Emulsifier, food coloring, nutrient, texturizer, thickener. Main high-quality, complete (contains all essential amino acids) protein in cow's milk. Added to foods like cream, coffee creamers, processed meats, cheeses, and frozen desserts, serving in a number of functional roles. Imparts white color to foods. Note that it is found in "nondairy" foods like soy cheese. Milk-allergic individuals need to avoid this ingredient. May also contribute sodium if in the form of sodium caseinate. Individuals who are allergic and sodium-sensitive individuals should limit intake of sodium caseinate. Rating: A+

Cellulose gum. See Carboxymethylcellulose and Gums

Chlorophyll *(CI natural green 3, chlorophyllin)*. Antioxidant, food coloring. Green pigment found in plants. Used to provide color to cheeses, dairy drinks, preserved fruits and vegetables, soups, ice cream, sauces, pasta. Chlorophyllin is the stabilized form of chlorophyll made by adding sodium or copper to chlorophyll. Found in dietary supplements. May act as antioxidant. Rating: A+

Chlorophyllin. See Chlorophyll

CI natural yellow 6. See Saffron

Citric acid *(sodium citrate)*. Acid, antioxidant, emulsifier, flavoring agent, preservative. Natural, widely occurring, sour-tasting acid from plants and animals. Made by fermenting sugars and can be extracted from citrus fruits (especially lemons and limes) and berries. Gives flavor to beverages (typically soft drinks and fruit juices), ice cream, and candy. Helps to adjust pH balance of fruit-containing products (juices, jellies, jams), desserts, dressings, canned and frozen vegetables, and dairy and fruit products. Can assist in preventing fats from sticking together, as in ice cream. Sodium-sensitive individuals should limit intake of sodium citrate. Rating: A

CMC. See Carboxymethylcellulose

Cochineal extract *(carmine)*. Artificial coloring. Red food coloring made from the eggs of the cochineal beetle. Used to give foods like confections, meat, and spices a red, pink, or purple coloring. Carmine refers to the purified form of cochineal. It is not always clearly labeled on food products, and is often listed as a "natural" additive. Potential for both to provoke (severe) allergic reactions. Avoid if allergic. Rating: F

Confectioner's glaze *(resinous glaze)*. Glazing agent. Resin (oily substance) harvested from beetle secretions. Used as clear coating on candies. There is some debate as to whether some parts of the beetle are included in the manufacture of the final product. May produce allergic reactions in sensitive individuals. Avoid if allergic. Rating: D

Corn sugar. See Dextrose

Corn syrup *(corn syrup solids)*. Humectant, sweetener, thickener. Sweet syrup made by treating corn starch with acid or enzymes; if dried, can be used as a solid ingredient (corn syrup solids) and added to powdered products like coffee creamers. Sweet due to its high content of dextrose, a form of sugar. When enzymes break down some of the dextrose in the corn syrup, the resulting product is called high-fructose corn syrup. Can be used to provide moisture and/or sweet flavor to a product. May cause allergic reaction in some individuals, especially those with corn allergy. Note that a food that contains this additive would most likely be a low-nutrient food (for example, beverages, cake, candy, imitation dairy substitutes). May be flavored with vanilla extract. When branched corn syrup (made by treating indigestible dextrin with hydrochloric acid) was fed to humans, diarrhea was experienced in two out of five men, but not noted in women. Avoid if allergic. Rating: C

Cottonseed oil. Emulsifier, texturizer. Oil made from seeds of the cotton plant. Processing of the oil involves removing pesticides. Downside for cotton crops is the high level of pesticides used on them and that they tend to be GMO (See

Genetically modified organisms under Hot Topics on p. 23). Commonly added to snack foods like potato chips. High in inflammatory (omega-6) polyunsaturated fats. Often hydrogenated to form a more solid oil (which results in production of trans fat). Rating: F

Cream of tartar. See Tartaric acid

Crocetin. See Saffron

Crocin. See Saffron

Dextrins *(maltodextrin)*. Stabilizer, sweetener, thickener. A water-soluble white or yellow powder consisting of short fragments of carbohydrates made from the breakdown of starch by acid and heat. Easily digested and sweet tasting because they are small chains of glucose, but some dextrins are chemically processed to be resistant to digestion. These forms of dextrins act as fiber, slowing the release of sugar into the bloodstream. Used extensively in numerous products (baked goods, beverages, gravies, pie fillings, puddings, soups) due to its safety and low cost. A common dextrin is maltodextrin, or corn-starch-derived fragments with no more than twenty glucose units. Dextrins can be made from rice, corn, potato, and tapioca. Some dextrins are derived from wheat—those avoiding gluten should avoid. May cause allergic reactions if sensitive to the source from which it is derived. Avoid if allergic. Rating: A

Dextrose *(glucose, corn sugar)*. Sweetener. Simple sugar compound found in living organisms. Occurs naturally in honey and fruits, and can be added to foods to supply additional sweetness. Derived from starch from various plants, usually corn. Diabetics and those with poor glucose control should monitor how much of this simple sugar they eat, since it can cause blood-sugar spikes. Americans eat too much of this refined sugar. May be beneficial for athletes in the form of quick-energy foods. Avoid if allergic. Rating: C

Diacetyl. Flavoring agent. A clear yellow-green liquid with a buttery odor that naturally occurs in products like alcoholic beverages, coffee, cheese, cocoa, and berries, but can also be made through fermentation of glucose. Used in a number of products to carry flavors—particularly microwave popcorn, margarines, and oils—to impart the aroma of butter. The U.S. National Institute for Occupational Safety and Health has determined that, when used as an artificial butter flavoring, it can be a respiratory hazard when heated to high temperatures and inhaled, such as in a factory setting. Most likely due to the number of lawsuits and publicity this additive has received in the past five to seven years, various food manufacturers have decided to omit its use in products. Diacetyl compounds may be potential carcinogens. Rating: F

Diacylglycerol oil *(See also Mono- and di-glycerides)*. Emulsifier, fat. Fat that occurs naturally in small amounts in oils. Sold as a new, patented oil source derived from canola and soy oils. Can replace vegetable oil in baked goods, pizza, mayonnaise, snack bars, soups, gravies, meal replacements, and frozen dinners. There is interest in enhancing the diacylglycerol content of oil for its potential effects on blood fats and weight loss. In 2005, Health Canada assessed the safety of a high-diacylglycerol oil and concluded that there are "no human food safety concerns" with such a product. Rating: A

Dioctyl sodium sulfosuccinate. Emulsifier, humectant, stabilizer, thickener. White, waxy solid added to dairy-based drinks, cheeses, sauces, and beverages. Commonly found as an emulsifier in cocoa-containing beverages. Used as a stool softener since 1943. Based on extensive animal studies, considered to be relatively nontoxic. Rating: A

Dipotassium tartrate. See Tartaric acid

Disodium citrate. See Sodium citrate

Disodium EDTA. See EDTA

Disodium guanylate, disodium inosinate. Flavoring agents. Disodium salts of guanylic and inosinic acids. Used to provide a savory ("umami") flavor to noodles, snack foods, rice, vegetables, cured meat, and soups, often together with monosodium glutamate (see Monosodium glutamate). Individuals with gout or uric acid kidney stones should limit their intake of these purine-containing additives. Sodium-sensitive individuals should also limit intake. May cause allergic reactions. Rating: B

Disodium tartrate. See Tartaric acid

Dried maltose syrup, dried malt syrup. See Maltose

EDTA *(ethylenediamine tetraacetic acid, calcium disodium EDTA, disodium EDTA)*. Acid, chelating agent. Widely used food and cosmetic additive that binds metals such as manganese, iron, lead, and copper left in foods from processing. Sequestering metals in foods is beneficial, since non-bound metals can become reactive in oils, causing them to become rancid. Various forms of EDTA are used to promote color and flavor retention in pickled cabbage, canned foods like carbonated soft drinks, vegetables, seafood, and beans, as well as alcoholic beverages, sauces, salad dressings, and sandwich spreads. Also used therapeutically by healthcare professionals for chelation therapy. Toxicity studies in animals indicate the lowest dose to cause a toxic effect is 750 milligrams per kilogram of body weight given daily. In lab animals, it has been found to be toxic to cells and genes, but not cancer causing. Acceptable daily intake (for calcium disodium EDTA) established for humans at 0–2.5 milligrams per kilogram body weight. Sodium-sensitive individuals should limit sodium forms of EDTA. Rating: B

Equal®. See Aspartame

Erythorbic acid (erythorbate, sodium erythorbate). Antioxidant. White-yellowish, water-soluble, crystalline antioxidant derived from vegetables and produced from sucrose. Used as an antioxidant in meat, dairy products, processed fruit, dried and canned vegetables, cereals, egg products, artificial sweeteners, condiments, soups, beverages, and baked goods. Similar in structure to, but not a substitute for, ascorbic acid (vitamin C). Eating it does not interact with vitamin C in the body, as demonstrated by University of Alabama researchers. Has been shown to promote iron absorption in humans in ways similar to vitamin C. Sodium-sensitive individuals should limit the sodium form. Rating: A

Erythritol. Bulking agent, humectant, sweetener. Naturally occurring sugar alcohol found in fruits and fermented foods. Manufactured by fermenting glucose using specific microorganisms. Found in low-calorie and diabetic foods. Like other sugar alcohols (see Sugar alcohols), bloating and diarrhea can result when ingesting high amounts (more than 10 grams daily). Rating: C

Ethylenediamine tetraacetic acid. See EDTA

Ethyl vanillin. See Vanillin

Evaporated cane juice. Sweetener. Sweetener made from unrefined, minimally processed juice from sugar cane. It may be easy to overlook on an ingredient label as a sweetener. The perception in the natural-food industry is that it is a "healthier" sugar, and a side-by-side nutrient analysis indicates it may contain just a few more vitamins and minerals, but not enough to make a difference in health measures. Sometimes comes as "organic." Seen as a better source of sugar due to less processing. However, it is still sugar. Rating: C

FD&C Blue No. 1. See Artificial colorings

FD&C Blue No. 2. See Artificial colorings

FD&C Green No. 3. See Artificial colorings

FD&C Red No. 3. See Artificial colorings

FD&C Red No. 40. See Artificial colorings

FD&C Yellow No. 6. See Artificial colorings

Ferric ammonium citrate. Anti-caking agent, nutrient. A source of iron that can be used as a dietary supplement. Found as an anti-caking agent in salt. Rating: A+

Ferric citrate *(ferrous citrate)*. Nutrient. Added to foods as a source of iron. Rating: A+

Ferrous fumarate. Nutrient. Added to foods as a source of iron. Rating: A+

Ferrous gluconate. Food coloring, nutrient. Used as a source of iron in foods and as a black colorant to create a rich, black color in olives. Rating: A+

Ferric phosphate. Nutrient. Added to foods as a source of iron. Rating: A+

Ferric pyrophosphate. Nutrient. Added to foods as a source of iron. Rating: A+

Fibersol-2. Nutrient. Soluble fiber made from cornstarch found in beverages, baked goods, meal replacements, energy bars, dairy-based products (yogurts, ice cream), cereals, sweeteners, snack foods, and processed meats. Like other fibers, reduces blood glucose levels, so may be beneficial for diabetics. Made from corn, so may provoke allergic reaction in individuals sensitive to corn products. Avoid if sensitive to corn. Rating: A+

Folic acid. Nutrient. A water-soluble B vitamin that occurs naturally in foods like leafy green vegetables. Can be taken in supplemental form. Needed especially by women before and during early pregnancy to prevent neural tube defects. Together with vitamins B6 and B12, may assist in reducing blood levels of homocysteine, a marker associated with heart-disease risk. The typical Recommended Daily Allowance (RDA) for adults with no special needs (like pregnancy) is 400 micrograms. Commonly found in enriched flours, breads, infant formulas, and ready-to-eat breakfast cereals. Rating: A+

Formic acid *(methanoic acid)*. Flavoring agent, preservative. Naturally occurring acid in metabolic processes in the human body. Present in ants, fruits, honey. Added as an antimicrobial to livestock feed and as a food additive to sauces, ice cream, sweet baked goods, and beverages. Rating: A

Fructose. Sweetener. Fructose, a sugar found naturally in fruit, can be added in dried, crystalline form to food products to enhance sweet taste. It is appealing since it has a low glycemic index (won't cause blood sugar to spike), so people with poor blood-glucose control may benefit by eating it. There exists a small percentage of individuals who may be sensitive to fructose. At high levels in the diet, they may respond negatively with increased blood fats and uric acid, and changes in appetite hormones that can lead to weight gain. There is a compositional difference between crystalline fructose (pure fructose) and high-fructose corn syrup (HFCS, which is made from cornstarch and contains glucose and other sugars in addition to fructose. See High-fructose corn syrup). However, often research on HFCS is incorrectly applied to crystalline fructose. High amounts of HFCS are found in processed, nutrient-poor foods. Fructose occurs in smaller amounts in foods. Fructose has milder effects on blood glucose and insulin than high-fructose corn syrup. Avoid if sensitive to fructose. Rating: B

Fumaric acid. Acid. Found in plants (for example, mushrooms and lichen) and as a key component of metabolism in animals and humans. Used since 1943 as a food additive. Nontoxic. Like other acids (for example, citric and tartaric acids), adds acidity and tartness to foods like powdered drinks, pie fillings, candy, and desserts. Rating: A

Furcelleran gum. See Gums

Gelatin. Emulsifier, gelling agent, stabilizer, thickener. Protein extracted by heating collagen found in bones, hide, hooves, connective tissues, and organs of animals (pigs, cows, fish, horses). Not a complete protein, since it lacks the amino acid tryptophan and contains only small amounts of methionine. Found in dry gelatin desserts, sausage casings, ice cream, and beverages. Rating: A

Glucitol. See Sorbitol

Gluconic acid. Acid, chelating agent, leavening agent. Naturally occurring acid that is made in the human body as part of carbohydrate metabolism. Also present naturally in foods like wine, fruit, and honey up to 1 percent. Produced commercially and added to foods like cake mixes, gelatin desserts, and beverages. Due to its acidic nature, it has a tangy taste, but is not as sour as other acids. Rating: A

Glucono delta-lactone. Acid, chelating agent, leavening agent. Naturally occurring acid that contains gluconic acid as part of its composition (see Gluconic acid). White powder commercially produced through carbohydrate fermentation and added to dairy products like cottage cheese and canned vegetables. Rating: A

Glucose. See Dextrose

Gluten *(wheat gluten)*. Dough conditioner, nutrient, stabilizer, texturizer, thickener. Principle protein fraction from wheat (can also be found in other grains, but wheat is most commonly used). Added to foods like breads, ice cream, and condiments for a variety of functions, but mainly to give structure and texture. Individuals with celiac disease need to follow a gluten-free diet. A gluten-free diet may also be helpful for those who are gluten intolerant but do not necessarily have celiac disease. (See Gluten under Hot Topics on p. 22). Due to the high number of individuals with gluten intolerance, it may be best to avoid this additive. Rating: F

Glycerin *(glycerine, glycerol)*. Humectant, sweetener, thickener. Provides the structural backbone for naturally occurring fats (triglycerides). Made from fat or synthetically manufactured by breaking down either carbohydrate or propylene. Synthetic forms are biologically similar to the natural form from fat. Used to make a source of energy, glycogen, in the body. Slight sweet taste (about 60 percent as sweet as table sugar). Used in a number of food products. Does not lead to rises in blood sugar or cause tooth cavities. Holds moisture in desserts, candies, and bars. Rating: A

Glycerol. See Glycerin

Grape color extract. Antioxidant, food coloring. A red-blue pigment composed of water-soluble antioxidants (called anthocyanins) used to impart color to grape juice and other beverages. Rating: A

Guaiac gum *(guaiacum, guaiac gum, gum guaiac)*. Antioxidant. Resinous antioxidant added to butter, margarine, lard, animal fats and oils, and sauces. Acceptable daily intake set at 0–2.5 milligrams per kilogram body weight. No effects seen in humans taking 50 or 100 milligrams daily for 18–104 weeks. Rating: A

Guar gum. See Gums

Gums *(Acacia, arabic, furcellaran, guar, karaya, locust bean, tragacanth, xanthan)*. Stabilizers, thickeners. Collectively, these are fibers from plant (seed, bean trees, seaweed) or bacterial sources. Acacia and arabic gums are the same ingredient—an extract from a tree source. Furcellaran is from red algae; guar and tragacanth gums are from legumes; karaya is from sterculia trees; locust bean gum is from carob seeds; xanthan gum is a bacterial fermentation product of sugars. Gums thicken candies, dressings, jellies, frostings, and cheeses, and stabilize beverages. May help delay the normal rise in blood sugar with eating, and may even contribute to satiety. Some gums are found in powdered laxatives. Since they swell with water, eating large amounts in laxative or fiber products without adequate fluid can lead to throat closure and difficulty breathing. Some individuals who may be allergic to the source of the gum should avoid it. Rating: A+

Hartshorn. See Ammonium bicarbonate

HFCS. See High-fructose corn syrup

High-fructose corn syrup *(HFCS).* Humectant, sweetener. Sweetener derived from corn, generally those varieties that are genetically modified. Corn starch is processed to corn syrup and then treated with enzymes to convert glucose into fructose. It can be further mixed with glucose corn syrup to alter the ratio of glucose to fructose. Typically, it is about half fructose (fruit sugar) and half glucose and tastes as sweet as table sugar. Commonly used in place of table sugar (sucrose) in soft drinks and other sweetened processed foods due to its low cost and how it functions in foods (adds moisture, makes for better browning). In a press release from *NutraIngredients.com* on April 2, 2008, the U.S. FDA was quoted as saying that products containing HFCS should not be labeled as "natural." Introduced in processed foods and beverages in the mid-1970s, it is thought that the increasing rates of obesity and diabetes are associated with HFCS intake. However, this is an area of active debate. Some individuals claim that these effects are not due to HFCS specifically, but to increased sugar intake overall. Rating: C

HVP. See Hydrolyzed vegetable protein

Hydrogenated starch hydrolysate *(hydrogenated glucose syrup, maltitol syrup, sorbitol syrup).* Humectant, sweetener. Sweeteners derived from corn, wheat, or potato starch by breaking down these substances into smaller fragments, followed by the process of hydrogenation (applying hydrogen gas under high pressure) to create a mixture of various sugar alcohols (see Sugar alcohols). Found in diabetic foods. As with other sugar alcohols, high amounts (10 grams or more daily) can have a laxative effect. Rating: C

Hydrogenated vegetable oil. See Partially hydrogenated oil

Hydrolyzed casein. See Hydrolyzed vegetable protein

Hydrolyzed soy protein. See Hydrolyzed vegetable protein

Hydrolyzed vegetable protein *(HVP, hydrolyzed protein, hydrolyzed soy protein, hydrolyzed wheat protein, hydrolyzed whey protein, hydrolyzed casein, TVP, texturized vegetable protein).* Flavor enhancer. Plant protein (often soy-based, but can be wheat- or corn-based—the source should be specified on the label) that has been broken down into amino acids. Incorporated into instant soups, meats, sauces, and beef stew because of its savory ("umami") meat flavor. Contains 10–30 percent MSG. Classified on some food labels as a "natural flavoring." May cause reactions like headache. Gluten-sensitive individuals should avoid if the source is wheat. Individuals with soy, wheat, or milk allergies should avoid proteins from these sources. Also avoid if allergic to MSG. Rating: F

Hydrolyzed wheat protein. See Hydrolyzed vegetable protein

Hydrolyzed whey protein. See Hydrolyzed vegetable protein

Iodized salt. See Salt

Iodized table salt. See Salt

Inulin. Bulking agent, (natural) fat substitute, fiber, nutrient, sweetener. Naturally occurring, slightly sweet fiber found in chicory root, garlic, leek, and Jerusalem artichokes. May be found in a variety of foods, from processed baked goods to more healthy fiber supplements. Considered to be healthy since it acts as a "prebiotic," or food for healthy gut bacteria, and also helps enhance calcium absorption. Has minimal effect on blood sugar; thought to be safe for diabetics. May cause allergic reaction in sensitive individuals, who should avoid it. Rating: A+

Invert sugar *(invert sugar syrup)*. Sweetener. A sweetener that contains half glucose and half fructose. More sweet and soluble than sucrose (table sugar). Produced commercially by "inverting" or splitting apart the sucrose molecule. Added to candy, confections, soft drinks, and a variety of other sweetened products. Rating: C

Iron phosphate. See Phosphates

Isoamyl acetate. Flavoring agent (artificial). Fruity flavoring that occurs naturally in bananas and pears, but is usually synthesized and used in beverages, ice cream, candy, baked goods, and flavored fruit sodas. Exposure to high amounts has resulted in headache, fatigue, increased pulse, and irritation of nose and throat. Rating: F

Isomalt *(isomaltitol)*. Anti-caking agent, bulking agent, emulsifier, glazing agent, sweetener. Sugar alcohol made from beets. Comprised of glucose and mannitol. Added to dairy-based products (cheese, milk powders, desserts), breakfast cereals, pastas, noodles, seasonings, condiments, and beverages. Found in low-calorie and diabetic foods, and blended with artificial sweeteners like acesulfame-potassium and sucralose. Like other sugar alcohols (see Sugar alcohols), bloating and diarrhea can result when ingesting high amounts (more than 10 grams daily). Rating: A

Karaya gum. See Gums

Lactic acid. Acid, preservative. Naturally occurring or chemically synthesized acid made by fermentation of milk carbohydrate (lactose), meat, and beers. Adds acidity to foods, preventing spoiling and enhancing tartness. Occurs naturally in the body and in foods. Can also be made commercially by fermentation of vegetable products like whey, cornstarch, potatoes, or molasses. Commonly found in dairy foods like cheeses, butter, margarines, and desserts. Used in fermented foods like pickles, beer, and sauerkraut. Rating: A

Lactitol. Bulking agent, humectant, sweetener. Sugar alcohol made from lactose (milk sugar). Lactose-sensitive individuals should avoid. Found in low-calorie and diabetic foods. Like other sugar alcohols (see Sugar alcohols), bloating and diarrhea can result when ingesting high amounts (more than 10 grams daily). Avoid if lactose intolerant. Rating: C

Lactose. Sweetener. Sugar from the whey portion of milk. Called "milk sugar." Used as a material for bacteria to ferment in the souring of milk. Included in cultured milk, dry powdered milks, eggnog, cream, and yogurt. Found in infant formula as a nutrient. Not as sweet as table sugar. Some people, especially Asians and African Americans, have a decreased ability to break down lactose—they are considered to be "lactose intolerant." They should avoid lactose to prevent gas, bloating, and diarrhea. Rating: A

Lecithin. Antioxidant, emulsifier. Compound consisting of choline (plays a role in brain health), fats, glycerol (see Glycerin), and phosphoric acid. Can be extracted from soybeans, corn, and eggs—often the source of lecithin will be stated on the ingredient list. Egg yolks are high (8–9 percent) in lecithin. Helps keep oils and water mixed together, reduces rancidity. Found in bakery desserts, chocolate products (milk chocolate). Some lecithins are "enzyme modified," or have the fatty acid in the middle position removed using an enzyme.

Enzyme-modified lecithin can be used in baked goods to extend shelf life. May be nutritious due to choline content. Rating: A+

Litesse®. See Polydextrose

Locust bean gum. See Gums

Lutein. Food coloring, nutrient. Yellow to orange-red powdered pigment found naturally in vegetables, especially corn and leafy greens like spinach and collard greens. Chicken feed is fortified with lutein to make the chicken's skin and egg yolks yellow. Added to a variety of foods like dairy products, pasta sauce, crackers, soups, egg substitutes, teas, cereals, soy milk, bars (for example, energy bars, granola bars), and beverages, and can be found in dietary supplements. Accumulates in the retina of the eye. Eating foods high in lutein may protect against blindness due to degeneration of the part of the retina called the macula. Lutein often occurs together with another carotenoid, zeaxanthin (see Zeaxanthin). Acceptable daily intake for either lutein or zeaxanthin separately or collectively is set at 0–2 milligrams per kilogram body weight. Rating: A+

Lycopene. Antioxidant, colorant. Bright-red plant pigment ("carotenoid") found naturally in red fruits and vegetables (for example, tomatoes and watermelon). Synthetic lycopene can be added to milk, yogurt, candies, cereals, baked goods, soups, salad dressings, and fruit and vegetable juices. Potent antioxidant. May play a role in preventing prostate cancer. Added to dietary supplements. Rating: A+

Magnesium *(magnesium aspartate, magnesium carbonate, magnesium chloride, magnesium citrate, magnesium gluconate, magnesium glycinate, magnesium oxide, magnesium sulfate).* Anti-caking agent, color stabilizer, flavor enhancer, nutrient. Mineral or mineral salt found naturally in a variety of fiber-containing foods including whole grains, vegetables, legumes, and seeds and nuts, as well as meats, dark chocolate, and coffee. Plays a role in the activity of many enzymes in the human body, especially those that affect the skeleton. Can be taken in over-the-counter preparations as a laxative. Recommended daily allowance (RDA) for adults is 400 milligrams for men ages nineteen to thirty and 310 milligrams for women the same age. The RDA increases to 420 and 320 milligrams for men and women ages thirty-one to fifty, respectively. Magnesium sulfate is commonly used as a flavor enhancer, whereas magnesium carbonate is known for its properties as an anti-caking agent. Added to dairy products or milk substitutes, cocoa powders, and salt for functional purposes and to a large variety of foods for its nutrient contribution. Can be taken in the form of a dietary supplement. Rating: A+

Malic acid. Acid, flavoring agent. Acid found in fruits such as apples, cherries, and grapes. First isolated from apple juice in 1785. Strong acid, imparts a high degree of tartness (think of a sour green apple). Added to fruit-juice concentrate, fruit juice, and fruit nectar. Rating: A

Maltitol. Bulking agent, humectant, sweetener. Sugar alcohol made from maltose, derived from corn syrup. Found in low-calorie and diabetic foods. As with other sugar alcohols (see Sugar alcohols), bloating and diarrhea can result when ingesting high amounts (more than 10 grams daily). Rating: C

Maltodextrin. See Dextrins

Maltose *(dried maltose syrup, maltose syrup, dried malt syrup).* Stabilizer, sweetener. Sugar derived from malt (barley is often the source). Made of two glucose units and only about one-third as sweet as table sugar. Can be fermented and thus is widely used in beers, cakes, and bread. Avoid if you are gluten intolerant. Rating: A

Mannitol. Bulking agent, humectant, sweetener. Sugar alcohol that naturally occurs in plants. Originally isolated from a deciduous tree (Flowering Ash) and referred to as "manna" after its similarity to the Biblical food. Found in low-calorie and diabetic foods. As with other sugar alcohols (see Sugar alcohols), bloating and diarrhea can result when ingesting high amounts (more than 10 grams daily). Rating: C

Methanoic acid. See Formic acid

Methyl vanillin. See Vanillin

Mineral oil. Anti-caking agent, glazing agent. Colorless, transparent oil that is a byproduct in the manufacture of gasoline. Added to cocoa products, confections, dried fruit, processed meat products, grains, fruits, and vegetables. Used medicinally as a laxative. Caused changes in lymph nodes when given to laboratory animals. Rating: C

Mixed tocopherols. See Vitamin E

Modified food starch. Emulsifier, fat substitute, stabilizer, thickener. Starch from corn, wheat, potato, rice, or tapioca that has been treated with chemicals so that its properties are optimized for a specific food application—for example, allowing it to perform under high heat or acid conditions. It can be made more digestible so it is included in foods that are easy to digest, like baby food. They are also used as thickeners in products like cheeses, sauces, pie fillings, gravies, and baked products. Concern has been raised regarding the chemicals used to modify the starch. Those who are sensitive to the starch sources named above should be aware that they may be sensitive to processed foods containing this ingredient. Rating: B

Mono- and **Di-glycerides.** Dough conditioners, emulsifiers, flavoring agent, stabilizers. Type of fat that has either one (mono-) or two (di-) fatty acids attached to a glycerol molecule. These fats are derived from animal and plant sources. May be made from oils (soybean, palm, cottonseed, sunflower) or chemically synthesized by reacting glycerin with fatty acids using an alkali agent. Works as an emulsifier in several foods (for example, peanut butter, margarine, and shortening). They give foods like margarine, breads, bagels, and baked goods a better consistency. Some, but not all, may be used in conjunction with a wheat carrier and tend to occur in nutrient-poor processed foods. Gluten-intolerant individuals should probably avoid. Rating: B

Monocalcium phosphate *(calcium dihydrogen phosphate)*. Dough conditioner, gelling agent, leavening agent. Acid that is used as a dough conditioner and leavening agent in breads, rolls, buns. When it reacts with an alkali like baking soda (sodium bicarbonate), carbon dioxide and salt are produced, providing leavening to baked bread products. Due to the presence of calcium, it can also function as a gelling agent in canned vegetables and fruit, and in fruit jelly. Rating: A

Monopotassium tartrate. See Tartaric acid

Monosodium citrate. See Sodium citrate

Monosodium glutamate *(MSG)*. Flavor enhancer. Sodium complexed to the amino acid, glutamic acid. Used to enhance savory ("umami") flavor in meats, sauces, spices, instant meals, and bouillon cubes. Some people are sensitive to MSG and may experience nerve-toxic effects like headaches, mood changes, numbness, nausea, weakness, and a burning sensation in the upper body. People who are sensitive to MSG may also encounter similar effects with aspartame/neotame. Natural flavorings, gelatin, hydrolyzed yeast, yeast extract, soy extracts, and hydrolyzed vegetable protein all contain glutamate. Rating: F

Monosodium tartrate. See Tartaric acid

MSG. See Monosodium glutamate

Naturlose®. See Tagatose

Neotame. Artificial sweetener. Similar in structure to aspartame. Contains aspartic acid and phenylalanine, like aspartame, but differs in that it contains a methyl ester. However, unlike aspartame, appears to be safe for individuals with phenylketonuria (PKU), since it does not metabolize to phenylalanine. Approved for use in foods, except meat and poultry, since 2002. Several thousand times (7,000–13,000) sweeter than table sugar and about 40 times sweeter than aspartame. In the past, not frequently used, but with concern about high-fructose corn syrup (HFCS, see High-fructose corn syrup), it is becoming a more popular choice. Found in soft drinks, bars, powdered drink mixes, juices, chewing gum, bread, frozen desserts, baked goods, and candies. Rating: F

Niacin. See Vitamin B3

Niacinamide. See Vitamin B3

Nicotinic acid. See Vitamin B3

NutraSweet®. See Aspartame

Olean®. See Olestra

Olestra *(Olean®)*. Fat substitute. Produced by Procter & Gamble; formed by the mixture of fatty acids and sucrose (called a "sucrose polyester"). It has fat-like properties, thus is used as a fat substitute. Approved as a food additive in 1996. Products containing olestra had to carry an FDA-mandated warning about side effects (abdominal cramping and loose stools) and had to contain additional levels of fat-soluble vitamins (A, D, E, K) due to their malabsorption. Studies have indicated that blood levels of dietary carotenoids (plant compounds like beta-carotene) are lower in people eating products with olestra. Subsequent evaluation of customer complaints resulted in the withdrawal of the initial labeling requirement on olestra in 2003 by the FDA. The Center for Science in the Public Interest opposes the use of olestra and accepts consumer complaints at *http://www.cspinet.org/olestraform/index.htm*. May be used in savory/salty ready-to-eat snacks (potato chips, tortilla chips, cheese puffs, crackers), tortillas, and ready-to-heat unpopped popcorn kernels. Does not get absorbed, so it has no calories. Long-term studies in humans are ongoing. It has been suggested that its consumption may worsen symptoms of irritable bowel syndrome (IBS). Rating: F

Pantothenic acid. See Vitamin B5

Paprika extract *(paprika oleoresin, capsanthin).* Flavoring agent, food coloring. Deep-red, sweet powder from dried pods of mild capsicum. The oleoresin (oily part of the plant) is extracted using approved solvents. Used as a spice and additive to color meats, confections, vegetable oils, and canned goods. Contains red pigment ("carotenoid"), capsanthin, which is fed to chickens to color egg yolks. Capsanthin is an antioxidant and may have some health benefit. High amounts (11 grams per kilogram body weight) found to be toxic in mice. Paprika belongs to the family of nightshade plants. Sensitive individuals should avoid this additive. Rating: A

Paprika oleoresin. See Paprika extract

Partially hydrogenated cottonseed oil. See Partially hydrogenated oil

Partially hydrogenated oil *(partially hydrogenated cottonseed oil, partially hydrogenated palm oil, partially hydrogenated soybean oil, partially hydrogenated vegetable oil).* Fat. Through the process known as hydrogenation, developed in the early 1900s, unsaturated vegetable fats can be made more solid and shelf stable. Crisco® shortening is a classical example of a hydrogenated-oil food product. As a result of hydrogenation, harmful trans fats are formed. Different types of trans fats also occur in small amounts in nature, such as in meat and milk. "Trans" refers to the chemical structure of the fat. Partially hydrogenated oil (and resulting trans fat) is found in a multitude of processed food items: dessert and bread mixes, pastries, cookies, donuts, cake, crackers, frozen meals, French fries, margarines, shortening, taco shells, and microwave popcorn.

Studies indicate that eating these fats have serious adverse health outcomes—probably more than any other fat, including saturated fat. They increase risk for heart disease by increasing "bad" (LDL) cholesterol and decreasing "good" (HDL) cholesterol. As a result of the available scientific data, the National Academy of Sciences has reported that there is "no safe amount" of trans fat. Other health effects relating to cancer, diabetes, infertility, and weight gain remain under investigation. A recent study published by researchers at the University of Rio de Janeiro found that, when lactating rats were fed hydrogenated oil at 11.75 percent of the total dietary fat, their offspring developed insulin resistance, or a condition in which, later in life, organs like the liver and muscle are no longer able to respond to insulin surges when eating. Most important, this study indicated that the negative effects of trans fat may span several generations. Since 2006, the amount of trans fat in a product can be found in the Nutrition Facts label under the fat category. Required labeling of trans fats has fueled food manufacturers to investigate substitutes for partially hydrogenated oil. Note that if the product contains less than 0.5 grams of trans fat it can be listed as "0 grams" on the label. However, if you read in the ingredient list that the product contains "partially hydrogenated oil," chances are it also contains trans fat. Rating: F

Partially hydrogenated palm oil. See Partially hydrogenated oil

Partially hydrogenated soybean oil. See Partially hydrogenated oil

Partially hydrogenated vegetable oil. See Partially hydrogenated oil

Phosphates *(calcium phosphate, iron phosphate, sodium aluminum phosphate, ammonium phosphate, sodium acid pyrophosphate, phosphoric acid, tetrasodium phosphate, tricalcium phosphate)*. Acid, chelating agent, color stabilizer, dough conditioner, emulsifier, firming agent, nutrient. Phosphoric acid is used as an acid and flavoring in bakery products, cheeses, beverages, candy, and dairy products. Phosphate is a nutrient and is needed in the body for kidney, intestine, and bone health, as well as for the proper functioning of the parathyroid gland (regulates vitamin D and calcium in the body).

Consuming too much, mainly by eating excessive meat and dairy products, can have adverse effects. A variety of phosphate additives are found in foods and have specific functions. Colas contain phosphoric acid as an acid. In a study by Tufts University, researchers found that women who were cola drinkers had low calcium-to-phosphorus ratio and a lower bone mineral density, suggesting that drinking large amounts of cola can lead to mineral imbalance in the body.

In addition to providing calcium as a nutrient, calcium phosphate is used in bread products, canned vegetables, and jellies. Tricalcium phosphate is often used as a supplemental source of calcium in foods like orange juice. Sodium aluminum phosphate is used in cheeses and together with sodium bicarbonate in self-rising flour. Tetrasodium phosphate suspends cocoa in milk. Ammonium phosphate is commonly found in baking powder and in bread products as a leavening agent. Sodium acid pyrophosphate provides different levels of leavening action in self-rising and prepared cakes, donuts, refrigerated dough, and other baking flours and mixes. It can be added to hot dogs and sausages to obtain a red color. Rating: A

Phosphoric acid. See Phosphates

Phytosterols/phytostanols *(plant sterols, plant stanols, stanol esters, beta-sitosterol, campesterol, stigmasterol)*. Nutrient. Cholesterol-like compounds found naturally in plant sources like vegetable oils, nuts, vegetables, and seeds. Ester forms are sometimes used in foods since they are more fat soluble. These beneficial additives reduce cholesterol absorption from food and lower LDL (bad) cholesterol in blood by 10–15 percent. Food products that contain these compounds in certain amounts are allowed to carry an FDA-approved health claim on heart-disease risk. A downside is that they may also slightly decrease absorption of dietary carotenoids (like beta-carotene). Commonly found added to margarine (Benecol®, Promise®), select juices, and salad dressings. Also found in dietary supplements. Rating: A+

Plant stanols. See Phytosterols/phytostanols

Plant sterols. See Phytosterols/phytostanols

Polydextrose *(Litesse®, Sta-Lite®, Trimcal)*. Bulking agent, humectant, sweetener. Ingredient formed by combining dextrose (from corn) with a sugar alcohol (sorbitol). Contains a small amount (1 percent) citric acid or (0.1 percent) phosphoric acid. Classified as a soluble fiber, it can replace calories, fat, and sugar in foods like baked goods, baking mixes, frostings, salad dressings, frozen desserts, sauces, and toppings. Tastes slightly sweet and is not fully absorbed. Laxation may be experienced when taking high amounts, similar to the effects of a sugar alcohol. A label warning must be included on a food product if a serving contains more than 15 grams of polydextrose. Rating: B

Polydimethylsiloxane. Anti-caking agent, anti-foaming agent. A synthetic ingredient made from silicone added to foods at levels of 10 milligrams to 110 milligrams per kilogram depending on the food category. Found in candy, confectionery, alcoholic beverages, fruit spreads, margarine, soups, canned vegetables and fruits, milk powder, chewing gum, and fruit-based desserts. Silicone implants have been shown to cause changes in the immune system of animals. Rating: C

Polyols. See Sugar alcohols

Polysorbate 60, Polysorbate 65, Polysorbate 80. Emulsifiers. Polysorbate 60's other name is polyoxyethylene (20) sorbitan monostearate. Polysorbate 65 and 80 are closely related and have other names as well: polyoxyethylene (20) sorbitan tristearate and polyoxyethylene (20) sorbitan monooleate, respectively. Each of them has slightly different emulsifying properties. The polysorbate trio can be used alone or in combination in a variety of products like whipped cream, cakes, cake mixes, cake icing, ice cream, frostings, powdered soft drink mixes, dessert mixes, and chocolate-flavored syrups. A study in rat intestines showed that polysorbates 60 and 80 led to a slightly more permeable gut. The authors of the study concluded that ingesting these additives may result in more toxic substances from foods getting into the body. However, there is no proof that this occurs. Cell studies have revealed that polysorbate 80 may change the response of immune cells and make cells more susceptible to oxidative stress (damage by reactive compounds). Rating: D

Polyvinylpyrrolidone *(PVP)*. Emulsifier, glazing agent, stabilizer, thickener. A polymer (substance made of repeating units) used to clarify beer, vinegar, and wine, and as a stabilizer in artificial sweeteners and dietary supplements (particularly in vitamin and mineral concentrates). Shown to be carcinogenic in laboratory animals when inhaled. No carcinogenic effects were noted with ingestion. Rating: B

Potassium bisulfite. See Sulfites

Potassium bromate. Dough conditioner. White crystals or powder used to improve the function of flour in products like bread, rolls, and buns. Also used for making fermented malt beverages or distilled spirits. Potassium bromate has been shown to cause cancer in animals and be toxic in human cells. Banned in Europe, Canada, China, Sri Lanka, Nigeria, Brazil, and Peru. Not banned in the U.S. If used in a product in California, label must carry a cancer warning. Some companies have removed potassium bromate from their manufacturing process. Present in a product if "bromated flour" is listed in the ingredients. Rating: F

Potassium carrageenan. See Carrageenan

Potassium caseinate. See Casein

Potassium chloride. Flavoring agent, flavor enhancer, nutrient, stabilizer, thickener. White solid powder that can be extracted from salt water or through separation of minerals. Can be used as a sodium substitute for table salt. Added to infant formula, dairy products, frozen desserts, vegetables, seaweeds, processed meats, egg products, cereals, pasta, noodles, beverages, confections. Needed in the body for acid/base balance, muscle contraction, and nerve function. Extremely high doses can cause heart symptoms, even cardiac arrest. Potassium-sensitive individuals should limit intake. Rating: A

Potassium citrate. Buffer. Potassium salt of citric acid. Used as a buffer in confections, jellies, preserves, and beverages. Rating: A

Potassium gluconate. Antioxidant, chelating agent. Potassium salt of gluconic acid (see Gluconic acid) made by glucose fermentation. Added as a white crystalline powder to dairy-based products (cheeses, cream, milk), vegetables (canned, dried), breakfast cereals, soy-based products, and beverages. Rating: A

Potassium iodide. Nutrient. Source of dietary iodine found in "iodized" table salt. High amounts can affect thyroid function. Rating: A+

Potassium metabisulfite. See Sulfites

Potassium sodium tartrate. See Tartaric acid

Potassium sorbate. See Sorbic acid

Propionic acid. See Calcium propionate

Propylene glycol. Anti-caking agent, antioxidant, dough conditioner, emulsifier, flavoring agent, humectant, preservative, stabilizer, thickener. Clear, thick liquid, also known as 1,2-propanediol, that does not occur in nature. A versatile additive, it is found in a wide spectrum of products, ranging from antifreeze and de-icing agents to paint and cosmetics. For food, the FDA allows it to be used at these maximum levels in products: 5 percent for alcoholic beverages, 24 percent for confections and frostings, 2.5 percent for frozen dairy, 97 percent for seasonings and flavorings, 5 percent for nut and nut products, and 2 percent for all other foods. Shown to be toxic when taken in large doses as part of various pharmaceutical preparations (e.g., intravenous administration). Rating: C

Propylene glycol alginate. Bulking agent, emulsifier, stabilizer, thickener. Yellow- to brown-colored grainy powder consisting of propylene glycol and alginic acid (see Alginate). In a clinical study, it was given to five men at 175 to 200 milligrams per kilogram body weight for twenty-three days without negative effects or allergic reactions. Found in a variety of foods including creams, spreads, noodles, processed cheese, and salad dressings. Acceptable daily intake set at 0–25 milligrams per kilogram body weight. Rating: C

Propylene glycol esters of fatty acids *(propylene glycol monostearate, propylene glycol stearate, propylene glycol diacetate).* Dough conditioner, emulsifier. White powder or viscous liquids made from propylene glycol and fatty acids. Found at various levels in foods like butter, margarine, dry cocoa mixes, dairy-based desserts, fruit fillings, cream powders, sugar syrups, pasta, noodles, and beverages. Acceptable daily intake for humans set at 0–25 milligrams per kilogram body weight. Rating: C

Propyl gallate *(propyl 3,4,5-trihydroxybenzoate)*. Antioxidant, preservative. White to cream-colored, slightly bitter crystalline solid additive chemically synthesized from gallic acid and propyl alcohol. Used in oils, meat products, chicken soup base, butter, margarine, breakfast cereals, desserts, and chewing gum. Prevents rancidity of fats. Commonly used in conjunction with BHA (see Butylated hydroxyanisole) and BHT (see Butylated hydroxytoluene). At high amounts (2.3 percent of the diet), short-term studies with rats led to death in 40 percent of the animals during the first month. Surviving animals showed retarded growth and renal damage at death. May be cancer-causing. Acceptable daily intake set at 0–0.2 milligrams per kilogram body weight. Rating: F

Pyridoxine. See Vitamin B6

Pyridoxine hydrochloride. See Vitamin B6

Quinine. Flavoring agent. Extract of the bark of South American cinchona tree used to flavor carbonated beverages (tonic water, bitter lemon) and alcoholic drinks (vermouth) in concentrations of up to 83 parts per million (83 milligrams per kilogram). Used as a pharmaceutical to treat malaria until the 1940s. Can also be used to treat leg cramps. Per FDA mandate, its inclusion in food and beverages requires prominent display on the label. May cause reactions in sensitive individuals. Some indications exist that it may not be safe for pregnant women. Avoid if pregnant or sensitive to quinine. Rating: D

Raw sugar. See Sugar

Retinyl acetate. See Vitamin A

Retinyl palmitate. See Vitamin A

Resinous glaze. See Confectioner's glaze

Riboflavin. See Vitamin B2

Riboflavin-5-phosphate. See Vitamin B2

Saccharin *(Sweet 'N Low®)*. Artificial sweetener. Saccharin, or 1,1-dioxo-1,2-benzothiazol-3-one, is 300 times sweeter than table sugar. It is the "oldest" artificial sweetener, having been used in foods for more than 100 years. Often blended with other sweeteners, since it may taste bitter or metallic at high concentrations. Added to beverages (fruit juices and drink mixes) in levels not to exceed 12 milligrams per fluid ounce. Used as a sugar substitute in individual packets. Processed foods may only have 30 milligrams of saccharin per serving. Causes bladder cancer in rats. There has been some debate about its cancer-causing potential in humans. Rating: F

Saffron *(CI natural yellow 6, crocin, crocetin)*. Food coloring. Yellow (or red-brown) powder from the *Crocus sativus* plant used as a spice and a food colorant. Crocin and crocetin are the pigments in saffron that give it its color. A report from the early 1960s describes a woman who ingested 5 grams of saffron along with estrogen tablets and experienced capillary damage in the skin and reduced blood platelets (needed for clotting). The dose considered to be toxic in mice is 20.7 grams. May have anti-cancer properties. Rating: B

Sal ammoniac. See Ammonium chloride

Salatrim *(Benefat™)*. Fat substitute. "Salatrim" stands for "short and long chain acyl triglyceride molecules." Modified fat developed from canola, cottonseed, soybean, or sunflower oils by Nabisco made of short fatty acids and a long fatty acid (stearic acid). Added to foods as a low-calorie fat substitute since 1994 (five calories per gram instead of the typical nine calories you get from fat). Does not get completely absorbed in the intestine like other fats. A recent study in twenty-two healthy, young men by researchers at the University of Copenhagen showed that, compared with traditional fat, salatrim modestly suppresses appetite to a greater extent. It did not change gut appetite hormones. Can be found in select reduced-fat cookies and chocolate chips. In large amounts (30 grams per day), may cause cramps and nausea. Rating: F

Salmiac. See Ammonium chloride

Salt *(sodium chloride, iodized salt, iodized table salt, table salt).* Flavoring agent, preservative. Sodium chloride, or common table salt, is one of the oldest known food additives. Iodized table salt is salt with added iodide (in the form of cuprous iodide or potassium iodide, added to prevent thyroid disease) and it may also contain an anti-caking agent to promote a free-flowing property of the crystals. Too much salt in the diet can lead to high blood pressure and increased risk for heart disease in susceptible individuals. Processed foods (frozen dinners, canned vegetables, and canned juices) contain relatively high amounts of sodium. Claims such as "low sodium" indicate that the food has 140 milligrams of sodium or less per serving. "Reduced sodium" implies that sodium has been reduced by 25 percent. The American Heart Association advised eating no more than 2400 milligrams of sodium (about one teaspoon) per day. The average American eats more than this amount (some sources cite typical consumption at 3300 milligrams per day). In late 2007, the consumer interest group Center for Science in the Public Interest petitioned the FDA to have stricter regulations on food sodium content. Sea salt (see Sea salt) is an alternative to iodized table salt. Rating: C

Sea salt. Flavoring agent. In contrast to table salt from rock sources, sea salt is evaporated seawater that contains a number of constituents (some valuable minerals) other than sodium and chloride. For example, sulfate, calcium, potassium, and magnesium give sea salt its unique taste. On the other hand, sea salt may also contain heavy metals from the ocean, including mercury, lead, and cadmium. Sea salt is often added to gourmet, high-end foods (for example, taro chips). There is ongoing debate as to whether sea salt is better than table salt. Rating: C

Sodium acid pyrophosphate. See Phosphates

Sodium alginate. See Alginate

Sodium aluminium phosphate. See Phosphates

Sodium aluminosilicate. See Sodium silicoaluminate

Sodium ascorbate. Antioxidant, preservative. A non-acidic form of vitamin C. Mineral ascorbates like sodium ascorbate are said to be better tolerated than ascorbic acid. Too much sodium ascorbate may result in increased sodium intake (see Salt). Commonly found in fruit juice and fruit nectar concentrates, as well as fruit juice and nectars, and meat. May also be added to numerous other processed foods. Sodium-sensitive individuals should limit their intake. Rating: A

Sodium benzoate *(benzoic acid)*. Preservative. Sodium benzoate is a chemically synthesized preservative used in soft drinks, fruit juices and preserves, jams, and margarine. Benzoic acid can occur in foods (plant and animal products) naturally, and at levels that are lower than typically needed in food for preservative action (40 milligrams per kilogram food versus 2000 milligrams of benzoic acid or sodium benzoate added to foods for their preservative quality). In animal studies, high amounts caused damage to the nervous system and brain. Sensitive individuals may develop hives or other allergic reactions. May encourage hyperactivity or decreased intellect in susceptible children. The Joint FAO/WHO Expert Committee on Food Additives (JECFA) has set an Acceptable Daily Intake (ADI) for humans at 0–5 milligrams per kilogram body weight. Sodium benzoate plus ascorbic acid can react under the right heat and light conditions to form benzene, a cancer-causing agent. Due to all the press generated on benzene's risks, soft drink companies are looking at substitutes to sodium benzoate. Rating: D

Sodium bicarbonate. See Baking soda

Sodium bisulfite. See Sulfites

Sodium carbonate *(washing soda, soda ash)*. Anti-caking agent, buffer, leavening agent, stabilizer. Sodium salt of carbonic acid. This white alkaline powder is added to breads, baked goods, noodles, pastas, confections, ice cream, and numerous other products. Contains sodium, so sodium-sensitive individuals should limit intake. Rating: A

Sodium carboxymethylcellulose. See Carboxymethylcellulose

Sodium carrageenan. See Carrageenan

Sodium caseinate. See Casein

Sodium chloride. See Salt

Sodium citrate *(monosodium citrate, disodium citrate, trisodium citrate)*. Acid, antioxidant, emulsifier, flavoring agent. The sodium salt of citric acid (see Citric acid) in the form of colorless crystals or white powder. All forms of sodium citrate contain sodium with trisodium citrate containing the most of the three. Therefore, sodium-sensitive individuals should reduce or avoid these compounds (see Salt). Some of these compounds (especially trisodium citrate) taste both sour and salty and are sometimes used to give products flavor (for example, club soda). Citrates can be also be used to emulsify fat—in ice cream, for example. Found within a broad spectrum of foods: dairy-based drinks, condensed milk, cheeses, margarine, processed fruit, breakfast cereals, soybean products, processed meats, vinegar, sauces, soups, condiments, and alcoholic beverages. Sodium-sensitive individuals should limit intake. Rating: C

Sodium erythorbate. See Erythorbic acid

Sodium gluconate. Chelating agent. Sodium salt of gluconic acid (see Gluconic acid) produced commercially by glucose fermentation. A fine, white crystalline powder added to dairy-based products (cheeses, margarine, frozen desserts), breakfast cereals, grain products (noodles, pastas), rice cakes, soy-based products. Contains sodium, so sodium-sensitive individuals should limit intake. Rating: A

Sodium hexametaphosphate *(sodium polymetaphosphate, Graham's salt)*. Emulsifier, sequestrant, texturizer. Sodium salt with high phosphate content. Note that high phosphate intake may lead to imbalance between other minerals in the body, such as calcium and magnesium. In 1975, animal studies on this additive indicated toxicity at doses up to 370 milligrams per kilogram body weight in mice and 240 milligrams per kilogram body weight in rats. Added to breakfast cereals, cake, fish, ice cream, beverages, puddings, and jellies. Used in water treatment—may be found in bottled water. May cause allergic reaction. Sodium- and phosphate-sensitive individuals should limit intake. Rating: C

Sodium hydrogen carbonate. See Baking soda

Sodium metabisulfite. See Sulfites

Sodium nitrate, sodium nitrite. Flavoring agent, food coloring, preservative. Sodium nitrate is the sodium salt of nitric acid, often appearing in the form of clear, colorless crystals. Similarly, sodium nitrite is the sodium salt of nitrous acid and comes as a white to yellowish powder. Both compounds are commonly used to preserve color in fish and meats, or keep them pink/red instead of brown. Sodium nitrite has replaced much of sodium nitrate use. These compounds also prevent the growth of bacteria like *Clostridium botulinium,* which is responsible for botulism. Sodium nitrate has been shown to be toxic in mammals. A single dose of one gram is toxic to humans; eight grams may be fatal and ingestion of thirteen to fifteen grams is generally fatal. Numerous cases of nitrate toxicity, especially in vulnerable populations like infants, have been documented due to contamination of well water with nitrate fertilizers. Nitrites and nitrates occur in vegetable sources such as root vegetables and leafy greens, especially when fertilizer is used.

In the presence of heat and amino acids (building blocks of protein), as in cooking meat or in the gastrointestinal tract, these compounds can form cancer-causing agents called N-nitrosamines. N-nitrosamines have been associated with migraines. Food companies have started to add acid (ascorbic acid or erythorbic acid) to meats to prevent nitrosamines from forming. In general, there are studies indicating that meat consumption may not be healthy. Specifically, studies demonstrating a link between colon cancer and meat consumption may suggest that sodium nitrite is involved. There is also some evidence that eating meats containing nitrites may lead to a lung disease (COPD). Various sources recommend that children and pregnant women avoid these compounds, as nitrites can cross the placenta. Rating: F

Sodium polymetaphosphate. See Sodium hexametaphosphate

Sodium potassium tartrate. See Tartaric acid

Sodium propionate. See Calcium propionate

Sodium silicoaluminate *(sodium aluminosilicate, aluminum sodium salt, aluminosilicic acid, aluminum sodium silicate).* Anti-caking agent. Fine, white crystalline solid that promotes the free flow of table salt and dried egg-yolk products at a level not to exceed 2 percent. This additive contains both sodium and aluminum. The association of aluminum with Alzheimer's disease remains inconclusive. Avoid aluminum-containing additives, however, in case of chronic renal disease, as there can be an accumulation of aluminum. Sodium silicate and magnesium trisilicate have been shown to produce damage in dog kidneys. Sodium-sensitive individuals should limit intake. Rating: F

Sodium sorbate. See Sorbic acid

Sodium stearoyl fumarate. See Calcium stearoyl lactate

Sodium stearoyl lactate. See Calcium stearoyl lactate

Sodium sulfite. See Sulfites

Sorbic acid *(calcium sorbate, potassium sorbate, sodium sorbate)*. Preservative. Naturally occurring preservative, first identified in unripe berries of *Sorbus aucuparia*, a plant grown in the northern hemisphere. Long-term feeding of 5 percent sorbic acid to rats resulted in no negative effects. Prevents mold, yeast, and bacterial growth. Sodium, calcium, or potassium salts of sorbic acid are used for their high water solubility. Overall, sorbates are used in a wide array of food (and cosmetic) products. Sodium-sensitive individuals should limit sodium forms. Rating: A

Sorbitan monostearate *(Span 60)*. Emulsifier. Waxy, creamy white powder synthesized by mixing fats together with sorbitol (see Sugar alcohols). Close relative of the polysorbates (see Polysorbate 60/80/85) and often used together with them. Incorporated into whipping cream, cakes, icings, cake mixes, puddings, etc. Tested in children and adults up to 4 and 6 grams per day respectively, and no harmful effects were noted after short-term use of about a month. Acceptable daily intake is set at 0–25 milligrams per kilogram body weight. Rating: B

Sorbitol *(glucitol)*. Bulking agent, humectant, sweetener. Sugar alcohol naturally found in fruits like berries, but can also be made by adding hydrogen (through hydrogenation) to the glucose molecule. Found in low-calorie and diabetic foods like candy, cough drops, jams, jellies, and baked goods. Like other sugar alcohols (see Sugar alcohols), bloating and diarrhea can result when ingesting high amounts (more than 10 grams daily). It has been suggested that its consumption may worsen symptoms of irritable bowel syndrome (IBS). Rating: C

Span 60. See Sorbitan monostearate

Splenda™. See Sucralose

Sta-Lite®. See Polydextrose

Stanol esters. See Phytosterols/phytostanols

Sterol esters. See Phytosterols/phytostanols

Stevia. Sweetener. "Stevia" refers to a large plant family, specifically to *Stevia rebaudiana Bertoni*, also known as sweetleaf. Very intensely sweet, it has been claimed to be 300 times sweeter than sugar. Available in the U.S. as a dietary supplement. There are mixed results on stevia: an older study found that it was weakly mutagenic (caused changes to DNA), while newer studies suggest that it may have health benefits like improving blood-sugar response. Recent work indicates it may actually protect DNA and improve immune system functioning. In 2006, the World Health Organization concluded that it was not toxic to genes and did not find evidence that it is a cancer-causing agent. Used extensively for more than thirty years in countries like Japan and in South America. Rating: A

Stigmasterol. See Phytosterols/phytostanols

Succinic acid. Acid, flavoring agent. Colorless, crystalline acid added to meats, condiments, and relishes. Found naturally in plant and animal tissues as a part of metabolism. A byproduct of sugar fermentation. Rating: A

Sucralose *(Splenda®)*. Artificial sweetener. Sucralose has many names: 1,6-dichloro-1,6-dideoxy-ß-D-fructofuranosyl-4-chloro-4-deoxy-α-D-galactopyranoside, 1',4,6'-trichlorogalactosucrose, trichlorosucrose, and Splenda®. Sucralose is chlorinated sucrose (3 chlorine atoms attached to table sugar) and is referred to as a "chlorinated sugar." Discovered in 1976, but not approved for use in the U.S. until 1998. Splenda® is prepared with added corn-derived fillers (maltodextrin and dextrose). These fillers are not always needed when added directly to food products like candy, desserts, and diet soft drinks. Used in several food items. More than 100 studies have been done on sucralose in the twenty years since its discovery that indicate it is non-toxic and doesn't cause tooth cavities. A human study concluded its safety in humans at amounts of 5 milligrams per kilogram per day when given for thirteen weeks. However, since it is a relatively new synthetic sweetener, no long-term studies have been done in humans. Although a large majority of studies indicate its safety, there have been some published case reports that it may trigger migraines. Sucralose appears to have adverse effects on the gut tissue. Research from a Japanese university demonstrated that sucralose caused DNA damage in the gut of mice. More recently, researchers at the Duke University Medical Center showed that rats fed sucralose at an equivalent acceptable dosage for humans as determined by the U.S. FDA experienced a reduction in beneficial gut bacteria. Rating: F

Sucrose. See Sugar

Sugar *(sucrose, table sugar, cane sugar, brown sugar, raw sugar).* Sweetener. Sugar, typically made from sugar beet or sugar cane, is not harmful unless large amounts are consumed over time. General dietary recommendations often include limiting consumption of foods containing sugars. International guidance from health authorities (World Health Organization and

Food and Agriculture Organization) suggest reducing free sugar intake (those added to foods and naturally occurring in fruits, etc.) to no more than 10 percent of total calories. Soft drinks, candy, desserts (cakes, donuts, pastries), baked products, and fruit juices are just some of the foods that contain relatively high amounts of sugars. According to survey results from 1999–2002 analyzed by the USDA's Human Nutrition Research Group (BHNRC), Americans are eating seventy-four pounds of added sugar every year, or about twenty-three teaspoons of sugar every day, which can lead to tooth decay and obesity, and, ultimately, to complications like Type 2 diabetes and heart disease. Choose natural sugars like fruit sugar (fructose) when possible and limit added sugar in all forms to as little as possible. Rating: C

Sugar alcohols *(erythritol, hydrogenated starch hydrolysate, lactitol, maltitol, mannitol, sorbitol, xylitol, polyols)*. Bulking agents, humectants, sweeteners. White, odorless, sweet powders that occur naturally in fruits, vegetables, grains, and fermented foods. They are not as sweet as sucrose, yet they are desirable because they are lower in calories. Since they are not well-absorbed, they have about 33–50 percent of the calories of sugar. Foods labeled as "sugar free" commonly contain sugar alcohols. For foods that contain relatively high amounts, additional food labeling stating that "Excess consumption may have a laxative effect" is required. Eating large amounts (above 10 grams per day) may have a laxative effect. Unlike sugar, sugar alcohols do not cause tooth decay. In fact, studies show that xylitol may be helpful in preventing cavities. When concentrated, some sugar alcohols produce a cooling sensation in the mouth (e.g, as in chewing gum). Some concern has been raised about ingestion of sugar alcohols and their effects on worsening irritable bowel syndrome (IBS). Small amounts in foods (less than 10 grams eaten per day) may be without effect for some individuals, but others may be sensitive to lesser amounts. Rating: C

Sulfites *(potassium bisulfite, potassium metabisulfite, sodium metabisulfite, sodium sulfite, sulfur dioxide, sodium bisulfite)*. Antioxidant, antimicrobial dough conditioner, preservative. Sulfur-containing compounds that can occur naturally in foods (for example, wine) or be added to foods (dried fruits and vegetables, dried potatoes, vinegar) as preservatives to help retain fluidity and color. Sulfites used to be added to raw vegetables, but were subsequently banned by the FDA in 1986 due to severe reactions. If added to foods at a level of 10 parts per million (or 10 milligrams per kilogram), a label declaration is required. Highly allergenic ingredient, particularly for those with asthma; can lead to migraines, hives, itching, and breathing difficulties. In particular, sulfur dioxide may be especially problematic. Avoid if you are allergic. Rating: F

Sulfur dioxide. See Sulfites

Sunett®. See Acesulfame-potassium

Sweet 'N Low®. See Saccharin

Sweet One®. See Acesulfame-potassium

Tagatose *(Naturlose®).* Sweetener. Naturally occurring sweetener found in dairy products, but can be produced commercially from milk sugar (lactose). Chemically, appears to be a close relative of fructose (see Fructose).Therefore, individuals who are fructose-intolerant should avoid tagatose. Some concerns were raised with initial data from rats showing increased liver, adrenal, kidney, and testes weights after taking tagatose. It may also increase blood levels of uric acid (risk factor for gout, a condition of joint inflammation) in susceptible individuals. It is only about 92 percent as sweet as sugar and has a little more than one-third of the calories. Permitted for use in foods in 2002. Acceptable daily intake was set in 2004 to be 0–125 milligrams per kilogram body weight. Individuals who are prone to gout or have difficulties metabolizing fructose should avoid. Rating: C

Tartaric acid *(monosodium tartrate, disodium tartrate, monopotassium tartrate, cream of tartar, dipotassium tartrate, sodium potassium tartrate, potassium sodium tartrate)*. Acid, firming agent, flavoring agent, humectant. Naturally occurring acid, found in fruits like grapes. Commercially synthesized as a byproduct of wine making. Found in its acid and salt forms in baking powder, jams, jellies, cocoa powder, wine, citrus dessert mixes, meat, and cheese products. Potassium bitartrate is also known as cream of tartar. Sodium salts provide sodium; therefore, sodium-sensitive individuals should limit intake. High amounts (several grams per day) can lead to laxative effects. Rating: B

Tetrasodium phosphate. See Phosphates

THBQ *(Tertiary butylhydroquinone, tert-butylhydroquinone)*. Antioxidant, preservative. Antioxidant used to prevent rancidity in oils and fats. Found in a variety of products, including butter, bread, confections, ice cream, margarines, pasta, and sauces. Often used in combination with other preservatives like BHA at levels of 100 to 400 milligrams per kilogram, depending on the food. Shown to be cancer-causing in animals. Rating: F

Thiamin chloride. See Vitamin B1

Thiamin HCl. See Vitamin B1

Thiamin hydrochloride. See Vitamin B1

Thiamin mononitrate. See Vitamin B1

Thiamin nitrate. See Vitamin B1

Titanium dioxide. Food coloring. Bright white, opaque pigment found in nature with versatile uses ranging from paint to food. Commonly found in personal care products like sunscreen and toothpaste. Food regulations require that it not exceed 1 percent the weight of the food. Found in dairy products, breakfast cereals, processed meat, condiments, puddings, salad dressings, and beverages. Inhalation shown to cause lung cancer in laboratory animals. Has not been demonstrated be a cancer-causing agent when consumed through food. Rating: C

Tricalcium phosphate. See Phosphates

Trisodium citrate. See Sodium citrate

Tragacanth gum. See Gums

Trans fat. See Partially hydrogenated oil

Trimcal. See Polydextrose

Turbinado sugar. Sweetener. Relatively unrefined sugar from the first pressing of the sugar cane that is lighter-colored than brown sugar due to its molasses content. Sometimes referred to as "raw sugar" or "sugar in the raw." Holds more moisture than table sugar and is slightly lower in calories. Rating: C

Turmeric *(curcumin)*. Antioxidant, food coloring. Bright orange-yellow pigment from the root of the plant, *Curcuma longa*. Can be chemically synthesized and added to baked goods, dairy products, curry powder, cooking oil, candy, breads, biscuits, crackers, salad dressings, soups, pickles, and margarine. Contains curcuminoids, which act as antioxidants and may have anti-inflammatory, anti-cancer properties. Rating: A+

Vanillin *(methyl vanillin, ethyl vanillin, vanillin acetate)*. Flavoring agent. Vanillin occurs naturally in the vanilla bean, along with hundreds of other compounds. Due to the expense and scarcity of the vanilla bean, vanillin, a synthetic flavoring derived as a waste product of the wood pulp industry, was developed. It is used in butter, ice cream, candy, baked goods, syrups, and liqueurs. Sometimes used together with vanilla. This combination extract is found on the food label as "vanilla-vanillin extract." Skin irritant. Acceptable daily intake set at 0–10 milligrams per kilogram body weight. Rating: A

Vanillin acetate. See Vanillin

Vanillylacetone. See Zingerone

Vital gluten. See Gluten

Vitamin A *(retinyl acetate, retinyl palmitate)*. Nutrient. Fat-soluble vitamin found in fatty animal products like eggs, meat (especially liver), milk, butter, and fish. Available commercially by extraction from fish oils or by chemical synthesis. Acetate and palmitate forms of retinol include a fatty acid (acetic acid, a short-chain fat, or palmitic acid, a long-chain fat) together with the vitamin A compound. There are many forms of "preformed" vitamin A, collectively referred to as "retinoids," with retinol as the most potent compound. Carotenoids like beta-carotene (see Beta-carotene) are vitamin A precursors, meaning that, once they are ingested, they convert to vitamin A. Vitamin A is used throughout the body, for vision, cell growth, bone development, immune function, and the structure of mucosal surfaces and skin. Recommended daily allowance (RDA) for adults is 900 micrograms (3000 IU) for men fourteen years and older, and 700 micrograms

(2300 IU) for women the same age. Different levels have been established for pregnant and lactating women. Taking too much (10,000 IU) for an extended period may increase the risk of osteoporosis and hip fracture in postmenopausal women and fracture in men. Excessive intake through vitamin A-fortified foods like margarine, breakfast cereals, and low-fat dairy products in conjunction with taking a vitamin A supplement may result in elevated serum retinol levels. Fat-soluble vitamins like vitamin A can be more toxic than water soluble vitamins due to their ability to accumulate in the body. Rating: C

Vitamin B1 *(thiamine, thiamin chloride, thiamin HCl, thiamin hydrochloride, thiamin mononitrate, thiamin nitrate, Vitamin B1)*. Nutrient. Water-soluble B vitamin found naturally in yeast, liver, whole grains, vegetables, and meats that is required in the body to metabolize carbohydrates and for nerve function. Recommended daily allowance (RDA) for adults is 1.2 milligrams for men fourteen years and older and 1.1 milligrams for women eighteen years and older. Ingesting large amounts of coffee and tea can react with thiamin in food, making it inactive. Added to fortified breakfast cereals, skimmed milk, enriched flours and grains, and enriched pasta. Can be taken in the form of a dietary supplement. Rating: A+

Vitamin B2 *(riboflavin, riboflavin-5-phosphate)*. Nutrient, colorant. Water-soluble B vitamin that naturally occurs in meat, eggs, vegetables, and milk. Prepared commercially from yeast. Can be synthesized from genetically modified yeast. Found in all living organisms, as it is required for cellular respiration. Indirectly involved in maintaining the integrity of blood cells. Recommended daily allowance (RDA) for adults is 1.3 milligrams for men fourteen years and older and 1.1 milligrams for women eighteen years and older. Added to a variety of fortified foods (baby foods, breakfast cereals, sauces, processed cheeses, breads, etc.) as a nutrient or as a colorant (it has a yellow-orange color). Riboflavin-5-phosphate, a more soluble form of riboflavin, is added to milk and other foods. Also found in dietary supplements. Rating: A+

Vitamin B3 *(niacin, niacinamide, nicotinic acid)*. Nutrient. Water-soluble B vitamin found in meat, grain, beans, vegetables, yeast, milk, and fish. Niacin compounds are used throughout the body to make energy and for more than 200 enzymes involved in energy-transfer reactions. High levels of niacin are available by prescription and as an over-the-counter supplement for high blood fats, although a common side effect is facial flushing. Niacinamide does not cause flushing, but doesn't have the same effect on blood fats. Starchy products like pasta, ready-to-eat cereals, rolls, buns, bakery products, macaroni, noodle products, and bread are commonly enriched with niacin, since it is one of the vitamins lost in processing. Recommended daily allowance (RDA) for adults is 16 milligrams for men fourteen years and older and 14 milligrams for women the same age. Rating: A+

Vitamin B5 *(calcium pantothenate, pantothenic acid)*. Nutrient. Water-soluble B vitamin found naturally in meat, vegetables, whole grains, legumes and milk, and can be added to breads, pasta, flour, dairy products, and beverages. In the body, used for metabolizing protein, fats, and carbohydrates. Recommended daily allowance (RDA) for men and women fourteen years and older is 5 milligrams. Rating: A+

Vitamin B6 *(pyridoxine, pyridoxine hydrochloride, pyridoxal phosphate, pyridoxal 5 phosphate, pyridoxal-5-phosphate, pyridoxamine, pyridoxine HCl, pyridoxine-5-phosphate)*. Nutrient. Water-soluble B vitamin found naturally in whole grains, vegetables, nuts, beans, eggs, and meat. Added to fortified foods like breakfast cereal, breads, pasta, baby foods, etc. and found in dietary supplements. In the body, used for metabolizing fats, proteins, and carbohydrates. Together with folic acid and vitamin B12, can help reduce blood levels of homocysteine, a compound associated with heart-disease risk. Recommended daily allowance (RDA) for adults is 1.3 milligrams for women nineteen to fifty years, and 1.5 milligrams for women older than fifty years. For men, the RDA is 1.3 milligrams for men fourteen to fifty years, and 1.7 milligrams for men older than fifty years. Rating: A+

Vitamin C *(ascorbic acid, ascorbate, ascorbyl palmitate, calcium ascorbate, L-ascorbic acid, sodium ascorbate)*. Acid, antioxidant, nutrient. Water-soluble vitamin naturally occurring in citrus fruits, and can also be chemically synthesized. Biologically necessary for humans for healthy teeth, bones, and blood vessels. Used as an antioxidant to preserve color of fresh and cured meats, vegetables, fruits, juices, etc. Can inhibit the formation of cancer compounds (see Sodium nitrites). Has been used since the 1930s to improve volume and texture of dough. Sodium ascorbate is a common form in drinks due to its ability to dissolve easily. Recommended daily allowance (RDA) for men nineteen years and older is 95 milligrams, and 75 milligrams for women the same age. Considered to be a safe compound at levels below 2000 mg daily. Rating: A+

Vitamin D *(cholecalciferol or vitamin D3; ergocalciferol, calciferol or vitamin D2)*. Nutrient. Fat-soluble vitamin often referred to as a hormone. Comes in a variety of forms. Food is most commonly supplemented with either ergocalciferol (vitamin D2, from yeast or fungi sources) or cholecalciferol (vitamin D3, from fish-liver oils), which is a more activated form of vitamin D than vitamin D2. Both these forms must be converted in the body to calcitriol (active form of vitamin D). Vitamin D can be found in eggs from hens supplemented with vitamin D-containing feed, oily fish, breakfast cereals and grains, margarine, calcium-fortified juices, and fortified milk. Assists in promoting bone health, together with minerals like calcium. May also play a role in cancer and autoimmune conditions. Likely safe below 2000 IU daily. Most fortified foods contain 100 IU vitamin D or less. Rating: A+

Vitamin E *(d-alpha tocopherol, dl-alpha tocopherol, alpha tocopherol acetate, alpha tocopheryl acetate, d-alpha-tocopheryl acid succinate, d-alpha-tocopheryl succinate, d-alpha tocotrienol, mixed tocopherols, palm tocotrienols, tocopherol, tocopherol acetate, tocopheryl acetate, mixed tocotrienols, vitamin E acetate, vitamin E succinate)*. Antioxidant, nutrient. A fat-soluble vitamin found naturally in vegetable oils, fruits, seeds, nuts, grains, eggs, and meat. Wheat germ is a notable source of vitamin E. The "natural" form of vitamin E is designated by the "d" (d-alpha tocopherol) whereas the "synthesized" form is indicated by the "dl" (dl-alpha tocopherol) before the name. The natural form is more available to the body than the synthetic form. Commonly added to fats and oils to prevent rancidity. Many of vitamin E's functions throughout the body may be related to its ability to serve as an antioxidant. Considered to be reasonably safe, depending on the dose added (levels above 400 IU on a daily basis may require medical supervision). Rating: A+

Wheat gluten. See Gluten

Xanthan gum. See Gums

Xylitol. Bulking agent, humectant, sweetener. Sugar alcohol naturally found in fruits. Added to low-calorie and diabetic foods like candy, cough drops, jams, jellies, and baked goods. Like other sugar alcohols (see Sugar alcohols), bloating and diarrhea can result when ingesting high amounts (20 grams). Rating: C

Zeaxanthin. Food coloring, nutrient. Orange-red powdered pigment found naturally in vegetables, especially corn and leafy greens like kale and collard greens. Added to a variety of foods such as beverages, breakfast cereals, egg products, oils, gravies, sauces, soups, candy, and juices. Accumulates in the retina of the eye. Eating foods high in zeaxanthin may protect against blindness due to degeneration of the part of the retina called the macula. Zeaxanthin often occurs together with another carotenoid, lutein (see Lutein). Acceptable daily intake for either lutein or zeaxanthin separately or collectively is set at 0–2 milligrams per kilogram body weight. Rating: A+

Zinc *(zinc chloride, zinc gluconate, zinc methionine sulfate, zinc oxide, zinc stearate, zinc sulfate)*. Nutrient. Essential element needed for more than 300 enzymes to work in the body, some of them responsible for making DNA. Also important for immune system functioning. High-protein foods like meat, seafood, nuts, legumes, and grains naturally contain zinc, but it can also be added to fortified foods like ready-to-eat breakfast cereals and beverages. Recommended daily allowance (RDA) for adults is 11 milligrams for men fourteen years and older and 8 milligrams for women nineteen years and older. Rating: A+

Zingerone *(vanillylacetone, 4-(4-hydroxy-3-methoxyphenyl)-2-butanone)*. Flavoring agent. A pungent flavoring agent used to flavor spice oils. Rating: A

Allergies, Sensitivities, and Other Special Considerations

This section contains information that can help you avoid potentially troublesome additives, depending on your food sensitivities, allergies, or other special considerations.

Potential Cancer-Causing Food Additives

Acesulfame-potassium (Sunett®, Sweet One®)
Artificial colorings
Aspartame (NutraSweet®, Equal®)
Butylated hydroxyanisole (BHA)
Butylated hydroxytoluene (BHT)
Caramel color
Carrageenan*
Diacetyl
Potassium bromate
Propyl gallate

---

* When degraded in the presence of high heat and fed in large amounts

Saccharin (Sweet 'N Low®)

Sodium benzoate†

Tert-butylhydroquinone (THBQ)

Additives that May Provoke Allergic Reactions

These additives may provoke allergic reactions like asthma, breathing difficulties, fatigue, headaches, increased heart rate, migraines, and skin reactions.

Agar

Alginate (alginic acid, algin, sodium alginate, Pacific kelp)

Annatto extract

Artificial colorings

Aspartame (NutraSweet®, Equal®)

Bromate (calcium bromate, potassium bromate)

Caffeine

Calcium propionate

Carmine

Cochineal extract

---

† In combination with ascorbic acid, may react under specific conditions to form benzene, a carcinogen

Gums (acacia, Arabic, furcellaran, guar, locust bean, tragacanth, xanthan)

Hydrolyzed vegetable protein (HVP, TVP, hydrolyzed soy protein, hydrolyzed wheat protein, hydrolyzed whey protein, hydrolyzed casein, texturized vegetable protein)

Inulin

Isoamyl acetate

Monosodium glutamate (MSG)

Neotame

Quinine

Sodium benzoate (benzoic acid)

Sodium hexametaphosphate

Sucralose (Splenda®)

Sulfites (potassium bisulfate, potassium metabisulfite, sodium metabisulfite, sodium sulfite, sulfur dioxide, sodium bisulfite)

Additives that May Cause Gastrointestinal Effects

These additives may cause gas, bloating, cramping, or changes in bowel movements.

Agar (agar-agar)

Alginate (alginic acid, algin, sodium alginate, Pacific kelp)

Carboxymethylcellulose (sodium carboxymethylcellulose)

Gluten

Gums (acacia, Arabic, furcellaran, guar, locust bean, tragacanth, xanthan)

Hydrogenated starch hydrolysate (hydrogenated glucose syrup, maltitol syrup, sorbitol syrup)

Inulin

Sugar alcohols (erythritol, lactitol, maltitol, mannitol, sorbitol [glucitol], xylitol)

Olestra (Olean®)

Polydextrose (Litesse®, Sta-Lite®, Trimcal)

Salatrim (Benefat®)

Vitamin C (high amounts have a laxative effect)

Additives Commonly Found in "Junk Foods"

Acesulfame-potassium (Sunett®, Sweet One")

Artificial colorings

Aspartame (NutraSweet®, Equal®)

Butylated hydroxyanisole (BHA)

Butylated hydroxytoluene (BHT)

Caramel color

Corn syrup (solids)

Dextrose

High-fructose corn syrup (HFCS)

Invert sugar

Neotame

Olestra (Olean®)

Partially hydrogenated oils (partially hydrogenated vegetable oil, partially hydrogenated soybean oil, partially hydrogenated palm oil)

Saccharin (Sweet 'N Low®)

Salatrim (Benefat®)

Salt (excessive amounts)

Sodium nitrate, sodium nitrite

Sucralose (Splenda®)

Sugar (sucrose, cane sugar, brown sugar, raw sugar) (excessive amounts)

Trans fat

Additives Lactose-Intolerant Individuals Should Avoid

All milk-containing products

Calcium (or Sodium) stearoyl lactylate

Lactitol

Lactose

Additives Gluten-Intolerant Individuals Should Avoid

Dextrins (wheat-derived: maltodextrin)

Gluten

Hydrogenated starch hydrolysate (wheat-derived: hydrogenated glucose syrup, maltitol syrup, sorbitol syrup)

Hydrolyzed vegetable protein (wheat-derived: HVP, hydrolyzed protein, hydrolyzed wheat protein, TVP, texturized vegetable protein)

Maltose (barley-derived: dried maltose syrup, maltose syrup, dried malt syrup)

Modified food starch (wheat-derived)

Mono- and Di-glycerides (wheat carrier)

Additives Sodium-Sensitive Individuals Should Limit

All additives with "sodium" in the name

All additives with "salt" in the name

Aluminosilicic acid (aluminum sodium salt, aluminum sodium silicate, disodium citrate)

Baking soda (bicarbonate of soda, sodium hydrogen carbonate, sodium bicarbonate)

Bibliography

Abou-Donia MB, El-Masry EM, Abdel-Rahman AA, McLendon RE, Schiffman SS. Splenda alters gut microflora and increases intestinal p-glycoprotein and cytochrome p-450 in male rats. J Toxicol Environ Health A. 2008;71(21):1415–29.

Alade SL, Brown RE, Paquet A Jr. Polysorbate 80 and E-Ferol toxicity. Pediatrics. 1986; Apr;77(4):593–7.

Anderson DM, Brydon WG, Eastwood MA, Sedgwick DM. Dietary effects of propylene glycol alginate in humans. Food Addit Contam. 1991;8(3):225–36.

Baird IM, Shephard NW, Merritt RJ, Hildick-Smith G. Repeated dose study of sucralose tolerance in human subjects. Food Chem Toxicol. 2000;38 Suppl 2:S123–9.

Brand-Miller J, Wolever TMS, Foster-Powell K, Colagiuri S. *The New Glucose Revolution: The Authoritative Guide to the Glycemic Index: The Dietary Solution for Lifelong Health.* Marlowe & Company, 2003.

Branen AL, Davidson PM, Salminen S. *Food Additives*. CRC Press, 2001.

Bray GA, Most M, Rood J, Redmann S, Smith SR. Hormonal responses to a fast-food meal compared with nutritionally comparable meals of different composition. Ann Nutr Metab. 2007;51(2):163–71.

Center for Science in the Public Interest. "Chemical Cuisine: A guide to food additives." Nutrition Action Health Letter, May 2008, p. 1–8.

Code of Federal Regulations, *http://www.gpoaccess.gov/cfr/index.html*

Codex General Standard for Food Additives (GSFA), *http://www.codexalimentarius.net/gsfaonline/additives/index.html*

Department of Health and Human Services, National Toxicology Program, *http://ntp.niehs.nih.gov/*

Dohoo IR, DesCôteaux L, Leslie K, Fredeen A, Shewfelt W, Preston A, Dowling P. A meta-analysis review of the effects of recombinant bovine somatotropin. 2. Effects on animal health, reproductive performance, and culling. Can J Vet Res. 2003;67(4):252–64.

Food Standards Agency, *http://www.foodstandards.gov.uk/*

Haas, EM. *Staying Healthy with Nutrition: The Complete Guide to Diet and Nutritional Medicine.* Celestial Arts Press, 2006.

Heller, L. "HFCS is not 'natural', says FDA," *NutraIngredients.com*, April 2, 2008. *http://www.nutraingredients-usa.com/news/ng.asp?n=84404-fcs-natural*

Houben GF, Abma PM, van den Berg H, van Dokkum W, van Loveren H, Penninks AH, Seinen W, Spanhaak S, Vos JG, Ockhuizen T. Effects of the colour additive caramel colour III on the immune system: a study with human volunteers. Food Chem Toxicol. 1992;30(9):749–57.

Houben GF, Penninks AH, Seinen W, Vos JG, Van Loveren H. Immunotoxic effects of the color additive caramel color III: immune function studies in rats. Fundam Appl Toxicol. 1993;20(1):30–7.

Houben GF, van den Berg H, Kuijpers MH, Lam BW, van Loveren H, Seinen W, Penninks AH. Effects of the color additive caramel color III and 2-acetyl-4(5)-tetrahydroxybutylimidazole (THI) on the immune system of rats. Toxicol Appl Pharmacol. 1992;113(1):43–54.

Huff J, LaDou J. Aspartame bioassay findings portend human cancer hazards. Int J Occup Environ Health. 2007;13(4):446–8.

Jacob SE, Stechschulte S. Formaldehyde, aspartame, and migraines: a possible connection. Dermatitis. 2008;19(3):E10–1.

International Programme on Chemical Safety, *http://www.inchem.org/*

Kishimoto Y, Wakabayashi S, Matsuda I, Fudaba H, Ohkuma K. Acute toxicity and mutagenicity study on branched corn syrup and evaluation of its laxative effect in humans. J Nutr Sci Vitaminol (Tokyo). 2001;47(2):126–31.

Lanigan RS, Yamarik TA. Final report on the safety assessment of BHT(1). Int J Toxicol. 2002;21 Suppl 2:19–94.

Lewis RJ. *Food Additives Handbook*. Van Nostrand Reinhold, 1989.

Lu C, Barr DB, Pearson MA, Waller LA. Dietary intake and its contribution to longitudinal organophosphorus pesticide exposure in urban/suburban children. Environ Health Perspect. 2008;116(4):537–42.

Maga JA, Tu AT. Food Additive Toxicology. CRC Press, 1995.

Metcalfe DD, Sampson HA, Simon RA. *Food Allergy: Adverse Reactions to Food and Food Additives*. Blackwell Publishing, 2003.

Natural Medicines Comprehensive Database, *www.naturaldatabase.com*

Natural Resources Defense Council, *http://www.nrdc.org/*

Nutrition Data, *http://www.nutritiondata.com/topics/food-additives*

Oregon State University, College of Health and Human Services, *http://food.oregonstate.edu/*

Oregon State University, Linus Pauling Institute, *http://lpi.oregonstate.edu/infocenter/*

Osso FS, Moreira AS, Teixeira MT, Pereira RO, Tavares do Carmo MG, Moura AS. Trans fatty acids in maternal milk lead to cardiac insulin resistance in adult offspring. Nutrition. 2008;24(7–8):727–32.

Purdue University, Center for New Crops and Plant Products, *http://www.hort.purdue.edu/newcrop/default.html*

Sasaki YF, Kawaguchi S, Kamaya A, Ohshita M, Kabasawa K, Iwama K, Taniguchi K, Tsuda S. The comet assay with 8 mouse organs: results with 39 currently used food additives. Mutat Res. 2002;519(1–2):103–19.

Sauberlich HE, Tamura T, Craig CB, Freeberg LE, Liu T. Effects of erythorbic acid on vitamin C metabolism in young women. Am J Clin Nutr. 1996;64(3):336–46.

Smith, JM. *Genetic Roulette: The Documented Health Risks of Genetically Engineered Foods.* Chelsea Green, 2007.

Sørensen LB, Cueto HT, Andersen MT, Bitz C, Holst JJ, Rehfeld JF, Astrup A. The effect of salatrim, a low-calorie modified triacylglycerol, on appetite and energy intake. Am J Clin Nutr. 2008;87(5):1163–9.

Statham, Bill. *What's in Your Food? The Truth About Food Additives from Aspartame to Xanthan Gum.* Running Press Book Publishers, 2007.

Swithers SE, Davidson TL. A role for sweet taste: calorie predictive relations in energy regulation by rats. Behav Neurosci. 2008;122(1):161–73.

Tagesson C, Edling C. Influence of surface-active food additives on the integrity and permeability of rat intestinal mucosa. Food Chem Toxicol. 1984;22(11):861–4.

Tatsuishi T, Oyama Y, Iwase K, Yamaguchi JY, Kobayashi M, Nishimura Y, Kanada A, Hirama S. Polysorbate 80 increases the susceptibility to oxidative stress in rat thymocytes. Toxicology. 2005;207(1):7–14.

Tucker KL, Morita K, Qiao N, Hannan MT, Cupples LA, Kiel DP. Colas, but not other carbonated beverages, are associated with low bone mineral density in older women: The Framingham Osteoporosis Study. Am J Clin Nutr. 2006;84(4):936–42.

U.S. Food and Drug Administration, Center for Food Safety and Applied Nutrition, *http://www.cfsan.fda.gov/*

U.S. National Library of Medicine and National Institutes of Health. PubMed, *http://www.ncbi.nlm.nih.gov/pubmed/*

Wageningen University, *www.food-info.net/uk*

Wikipedia, "Food Additive" *http://en.wikipedia.org/wiki/Food_additive,*"accessed 4/1/2008

Winter, Ruth. *A Consumer's Dictionary of Food Additives.* Three Rivers Press, 2004.

Wittenberg, MM. *Pocket Guide to Good Food*. The Crossing Press, 1996.

Yun AJ, Doux JD. Unhappy meal: how our need to detect stress may have shaped our preferences for taste. Med Hypotheses. 2007;69(4):746–51.

Consumer Resources

Center for Science in the Public Interest (CSPI)

A consumer watchdog organization in existence since 1972: *http://www.cspinet.org/*

Code of Federal Regulations (CFR)

Federal regulations set forth by the national government: *http://www.gpoaccess.gov/cfr/index.html*

Food and Drug Administration (FDA)

Food additive database: *http://vm.cfsan.fda.gov/~dms/eafus.html*

Institute for Agriculture and Trade Policy

The pulse on the intersection between policy and practice for fair, sustainable food growing: *http://www.iatp.org*

International Programme on Chemical Safety

Chemical safety information from intergovernmental organizations: *http://www.inchem.org/*

National Toxicology Program, Department of Health and Human Services

Evaluates public health concern using toxicology and molecular biology: *http://ntp.niehs.nih.gov/*

Organic Consumers Association

For those who want more information on how to be proactive in the organic market: *http://www.organicconsumers.org/*

PubMed

A free service of the National Library of Medicine providing access to over 17 million scientific citations: *http://www.ncbi.nlm.nih.gov/pubmed/*

U.S. Food and Drug Administration, Center for Food Safety and Applied Nutrition

Federal regulations around safety of food additives: *http://www.cfsan.fda.gov/*

Wageningen University, Food Science Department

Provides food allergy dictionaries in over 30 languages, comprehensive food additive listing, *http://www.food-info.net/uk/*

About the Author

Deanna M. Minich, Ph.D., C.N., is a nutritionist, educator, and author with more than fifteen years experience in the nutrition field, ranging from innovating products in the food and dietary supplement industries to counseling patients in private practice. Her first book, *Chakra Foods for Optimum Health* was published to critical acclaim in 2009. Currently, Dr. Minich lives in Port Orchard, Washington, where she writes and teaches on nutrition topics. See her website for more information: *www.foodandspirit.com.*

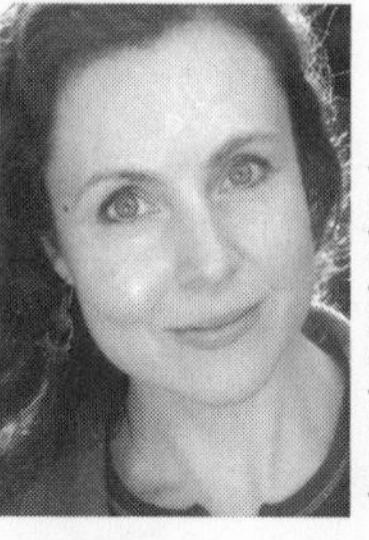

photograph © Mark Duhamel

To Our Readers

Conari Press, an imprint of Red Wheel/Weiser, publishes books on topics ranging from spirituality, personal growth, and relationships to women's issues, parenting, and social issues. Our mission is to publish quality books that will make a difference in people's lives—how we feel about ourselves and how we relate to one another. We value integrity, compassion, and receptivity, both in the books we publish and in the way we do business.

Our readers are our most important resource, and we value your input, suggestions, and ideas about what you would like to see published. Please feel free to contact us, to request our latest book catalog, or to be added to our mailing list.

Conari Press
An imprint of Red Wheel/Weiser, LLC
500 Third Street, Suite 230
San Francisco, CA 94107
www.redwheelweiser.com